DCU LIBRARY

080079121

WITH...

D1757283

Principles and Practice of Isokinetics in Sports Medicine and Rehabilitation

WITHDRAWN

Chief Editors

Kai-Ming CHAN

Nicola MAFFULLI

Editors

Pirkko KORKIA   **Raymond C.T. LI**

Foreword by Per A. F. H. RENSTRÖM

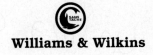

Williams & Wilkins

Publisher: Williams & Wilkins Asia-Pacific Ltd.

Regional Managing Director: George CIOFULI

Publishing Manager: Fanny F.Y. WONG

Editor: Chung-Lin NG

Editorial Assistant: Elaine Y.L. KONG

Copyright© June 1996 by Williams & Wilkins Asia-Pacific Ltd.

All rights reserved. No part of this publication may be reproduced, electronically or mechanically, including photocopying, resending or in any information storage and retrieval system, or transmitted any form, by any means, without prior written permission from the Publisher.

Williams & Wilkins Asia-Pacific Ltd.
Room 808 Metroplaza Tower 2
223 Hing Fong Road
New Territories
Hong Kong

Printed in Hong Kong

ISBN 962-356-016-8

617·1027 CHO

080079121

Chief Editors

Kai-Ming CHAN, OBE

MBBS, MCh (Orth)(Liv), FRCS (Glas), FRCS (Ed) FRCSEd (Orth)

Professor and Chairman, Department of Orthopedics and Traumatology,

The Chinese University of Hong Kong,

Prince of Wales Hospital, Shatin, Hong Kong

Nicola MAFFULLI

MD, MS, PhD, MIBiol, FRCS(Orth)

Clinical Senior Lecturer and Consultant Orthopedic Surgeon,

University of Aberdeen Medical School, Aberdeen, Scotland, UK

Editors

Pirkko KORKIA

BSc, MSc

Senior Lecturer,

Department of Sports and

Exercise Science,

University of Luton,

Luton, England,

UK

Raymond C.T. LI

MCSP, MPhil

Research Physiotherapist,

Department of Orthopedics and

Traumatology,

The Chinese University of Hong Kong,

Prince of Wales Hospital,

Shatin, Hong Kong

International Contributors

Todd S. ELLENBECKER
MS, PT, SCS, CSCS
Clinic Director, Physiotherapy Associates, Scottsdale Sports Clinic, Scottsdale, USA

Walter R. FRONTERA
MD, PhD
Associate Professor and Chairman, Department of Physical Medicine and
Rehabilitation, Harvard Medical School and Spaulding Rehabilitation Hospital,
Boston, Massachusetts, USA

William E. GARRETT, Jr
MD, PhD
Professor, Department of Orthopedic Surgery, Duke University Medical Center,
Durham, USA

Scott M. LEPHART
PhD, ATC
Director, Sports Medicine and Athletic Training;
Director, Neuromuscular Research Laboratory,
University of Pittsburgh, Pennsylvania, USA

Terry R. MALONE
EdD, PT, ATC
Associate Professor and Director, Division of Physical Therapy,
University of Kentucky, Lextington, USA

Tony PARKER
PhD, FASMF
Professor, Head, School of Human Movement, Faculty of Health Science,
Queensland University of Technology, Queensland, Australia

Danny M. PINCIVERO
MEd, BA
Doctoral student, Exercise Physiology/Sports Medicine,
University of Pittsburgh, Pennsylvania, USA

Per A.F.H. RENSTRÖM
MD, PhD
Professor of Sports Medicine, Department of Orthopedics and Rehabilitation,
University of Vermont, McClure Musculoskeletal Research Center, Vermont, USA

Christer G. ROLF
MD, PhD
Associate Professor and Head, Section of Sports Medicine, Department of Orthopedic
Surgery, Karolinska Institute, Huddinge University Hospital, Huddinge, Sweden

Joseph A. SALAM
Consultant Surgeon, Traumatology and Sport Medicine;
Medical Director for Rehabilitation Center,
Clinic for Surgery, Sport Injury and Arthoscopy, Heikendorf, Germany

Kent E. TIMM
PhD, PT, ATC, FACSM
Research and Development Specialist, St. Luke's Healthcare Association;
Leader, Athletic Medicine Team, St. Luke's Hospital OSF,
Saginaw, Michigan, USA
Research Consultant, Sports Medicine Division,
United States Olympic Committee

Foreword

Muscle strength is a major component influencing the performance in most sports. Many athletes therefore spend much of the time in developing their strength using whatever techniques and machines available. Since the concept of accommodated resistance that is the characteristic feature of the isokinetic devices developed in the end of the 1960s, the use of isokinetics is a valuable tool in the strength training program. It has with time been increasingly used as a testing device and for scientific evaluation of muscle strength.

A very important effect of the development of the isokinetic device has been its contribution to science. The use of isokinetic testing devices has been more or less the only reliable technique to make objective quantification of muscle strength. This muscle testing technique has been carefully validated through the years and has been shown to have great accuracy and reproducibility. Some of the first validation studies were made here at the University of Vermont. The isokinetic evaluation technique has therefore been extensively used in the last 25 years in hundreds of scientific studies. These studies have verified that isokinetic training is very effective and that it is one of the best ways to develop strength both at slow and fast speeds. It has also been shown that the training is rather selective.

As the isokinetic training is effective, athletes have not only used it in training, but, also in the rehabilitation after injuries. The concept of accommodated resistance means that this type of exercise is often reasonably well tolerated by joints and soft tissues. It is therefore a decreased risk for injury and for re-injury in the rehabilitation after an injury. Our group has even shown the isokinetic training to be effective in the training of amputated patients. The evaluation of muscle strength can also be used in prevention as existing muscle imbalances can be revealed and thereafter corrected and by that the risk for injuries will decrease.

As the isokinetic exercise and testing principle is used so extensively in both research and in exercise to increase strength, summarizing what we know scientifically about this valuable techniques is important. It is therefore of great value that the group from Hong Kong has taken the initiative to gather existing data of all the different aspects of isokinetics in one book. This book will serve as a very important instrument in the hands of teachers and lecturers in Sports Medicine at different levels of education. This book will be valuable not only for MDs but also for physical therapists, trainers, nurses, coaches, athletes etc active in Sports Medicine education and science around the world.

I would like to congratulate Kai-Ming Chan and his coworkers for producing this book that I am sure will be a great contribution in the field.

Per A.F.H. Renström, MD, PhD
Professor of Sports Medicine
University of Vermont, USA

Preface

The development and refinement of isokinetic technology has made objective quantification of muscle strength possible. Isokinetic assessment can be of major use in Sports Medicine in preventing, diagnosing and rehabilitating injuries, while in Sports Science it can be used to predict performance and to assess performance variables. Most work on isokinetics has involved the muscle groups around the knee joint, while the testing of other joints is less well validated. With recent developments in technology, reliable testing of other muscle groups, such as the trunk, has become possible.

Our interest in the isokinetic assessment of muscle function dates back into the early 1980s. Throughout this time, we have employed isokinetic techniques for research, clinical testing, rehabilitation and strength training of athletes. The major advantages of these methods have been their effectiveness, reliability, objectivity and noninvasiveness.

Principles and Practice of Isokinetics in Sports Medicine and Rehabilitation is a practical guide for isokinetic assessment. The scientific value of isokinetics is highlighted both for Sports Medicine and Sports Sciences. This will enable Sports Medicine practitioners to identify the merits of isokinetics and its relevant applications. The section on practical applications of isokinetics presents a step-by-step guide on the practical procedures necessary for accurate testing and a critique on the significance and validity of the variables commonly measured. Practical problems with testing and assessment are considered. The use of isokinetics in injury diagnosis and rehabilitation is outlined with specific illustrations from the research data collected at The Chinese University of Hong Kong. Assessment of the most commonly injured sites, including the knee, ankle, shoulder and the trunk is discussed. Guidelines are given on the interpretation of test results, and examples on how to apply them in designing appropriate rehabilitation programs are shown. A special section is devoted to the use of isokinetics in the assessment of sports performance.

The section Isokinetic technology: a global exchange provides the reader with the views of an international panel of distinguished authors on the value of isokinetics in research and clinical practice, and their thoughts on the future developments in this field.

This book documents the state-of-the-art of isokinetic technology and science and is intended as practical reference for professionals in Sports Medicine, Sports Science and Rehabilitation.

The Editors

Acknowledgment

We would like to acknowledge Mr. Raymond So, Ms. Josephine Yeung, Mr. Charles Lo and Dr. John S.P. Wong whose theses contributed to the scientific content of the book. We are grateful for the contributions of the international panel of authors and the message from Prof. Per A.F.H. Renström in the Foreword. Special tribute is also accorded to Ms. Sierra Choi, Ms. Amy Au, Ms. Barbara Chan and Dr. Vassilious Baltzopoulos for their clerical, proof-reading, liaison work and review in the preparation of this book. We would also like to thank the Hong Kong Sports Institute for their generosity of supplying us part of the photos in this book.

The Editors

ACL: anterior cruciate ligament

ACLI: anterior cruciate ligament insufficiency

AKP: anterior knee pain

ALRI: anterior lateral rotational instability

AP: average power

AST: angle-specific torque

BWR: best work repetition

CDRC: Cybex data reduction computer

CKC: closed kinetic chain

Con: concentric

CPM: continuous passive motion

CV: cardiovascular

DF: dorsiflexion

DOMS: delayed onset of muscle soreness

Ecc: eccentric

EE: elbow extensors

EF: elbow flexors

EMG: electromyography

EV: eversion

FT: fast twitch

HKSI: Hong Kong Sports Institute

H:Q: hamstring/quadriceps torque ratios

IEMG: integrated electromyography

IV: inversion

J: joules

KE: knee extensors

KF: knee flexors

MDH: malate dehydrogenase

MMT: manual muscle testing

MPT: mean peak torque

MRC: Medical Research Council

OKC: open kinetic chain

PCL: posterior cruciate ligament

PF: plantarflexion

PKF: phosphofructokinase

PKTAE: peak torque acceleration energy

PNF: proprioceptive neuromuscular facilitation

PP: peak power

PT: peak torque

PTW: peak torque to weight ratio

PW: peak work

ROM: range of motion

S: sprint

SDH: succinic dehydrogenase

SIR/SER: shoulder internal rotators/shoulder external rotators ratio

SSC: stretch-shortening cycle

ST: slow twitch

TEF: trunk extension/flexion unit

TEFTR: trunk extension/flexion testing and rehabilitation unit

TRTD: time rate of tension development

TW: total work

UBXT: upper body exercise table

Table of Contents

SECTION 1

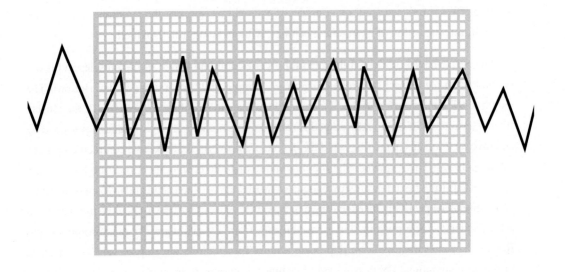

INTRODUCTION TO ISOKINETICS

I. Introduction to Isokinetics and Definitions

Dynamic muscle strength is quantified by measuring the force exerted on a system. Uniquely, isokinetic exercise involves a dynamic preset fixed velocity, with resistance varying exactly in response to the force applied by the individual, throughout a specified range of motion (ROM). This allows maximum resistance to be applied throughout the ROM, which is not possible with any other resistance training and testing appliance. For example, when lifting free weights, the load applied is restricted by the weakest point in ROM, and, consequently, the training effect is reduced at all other angles. To avoid this, some of the hydraulic training machines mimic the action of isokinetic machines, without being truly isokinetic.

The performance of a given muscle group varies with the length of the muscle, and is explained by the length-tension relationship (see Huijing 1992 for a detailed description). The length-tension relationship of the whole muscle reflects the mechanical behavior of the muscle fiber. The amount of tension developed is related to the number of cross-bridges between actin and myosin filaments in the fibers and the degree of the overlap of these two contractile proteins (Huijing 1992). This explains why the magnitude of force development must be less when a given joint is fully flexed or fully extended, as the overlap between actin and myosin is maximal and minimal, respectively. In executing a biceps curl, for example, the lift is often initiated from a fully extended arm position and, consequently, from a weak angle. As the arm moves into flexion, a greater degree of overlap occurs, more force can be developed, yet the resistance provided is unoptimal. With isokinetic machines, optimum resistance is provided at all joint angles.

Isokinetic techniques test a joint movement, for example the internal rotation of the shoulder, rather than the function of a specific muscle. Information on specific muscle activity may be obtained by simultaneous electromyography (EMG).

A. A brief history of isokinetic science

Isokinetic rehabilitative devices were developed in the late 1960s when the concept of isokinetic exercise was introduced by James Perrine. Since then, numerous studies have been carried out using isokinetic dynamometry. While isometric and isoinertial exercises play an important role in rehabilitation, isokinetic evaluation and exercises have attracted much attention because of the special features they offer. The most common dynamometers currently on the market include, for example, the Biodex (Biodex Medical Systems Inc.), the Cybex (Division of Lumex Inc.), the Kin-Com (Chattanooga Group Inc.), the Lido (Loredan Biomedical), and the Merac (Universal Gym Equipment Inc.) systems. Some of them are illustrated in Figure 1-1. The evolution of isokinetic machines has progressed steadily, with the refinement of functions and increased range of facilities helped by the advancement of computer science. In the late 1960s, isokinetic machines included a basic or simple computer program capable of comparing bilateral data, updated to enable the computation of total work, power and endurance. This was followed by the introduction of a monitor which provided immediate feedback to the therapist and the patient alike. More recently, touch-on monitors have been incorporated, with computers capable of more complex tasks, including the computation of fatigue index, displaying progress in the training program gravity correction and improved data storage capacity. Eccentric mode has been added as an option. Advancements in the provision of accessories have also provided more scope for muscle testing and rehabilitation. It is now possible to test all limbs, and recently, a trunk testing facility has become available which allows trunk flexion and extension, rotation and lifting, and closed kinetic chain exercise (CKC). All planes of movement can be tested, including proprioceptive neuromuscular facilitation (PNF) movements. Recently, machines have been developed specifically for muscle training, such as a stairclimber, cycle ergometer and a swimbench.

The development of Sports Medicine and Sports Science has made the accurate quantification of human muscle performance increasingly important. The measurement of muscle strength is vital in diagnosing muscle weaknesses, assessing specific injuries, and evaluating the effectiveness of a rehabilitation program (Sapega 1990). In Sports Science, the measurement of muscle strength is essential in the evaluation of the effectiveness of strength training programs, in identifying weaknesses as well as talent (Astrand and Rodahl 1986). Before the concept of isokinetic exercise emerged (Hislop and Perrine 1967), physicians relied on manual testing and static dynamometers which provided little information on the dynamic qualities of muscle action. Those who advocate the use of isokinetics in muscle strength testing feel that they offer greater measurement reliability and objectivity: they offer greater control over velocity of motion, technique and extraneous movement, and the assessment of strength and power can be made within one contraction (Abernethy et al 1995). The "skeptics" argue that the movements involved and the loading applied are artificial and are not related to movements that occur during sporting movements (Kannus 1994, Mahler et al 1992).

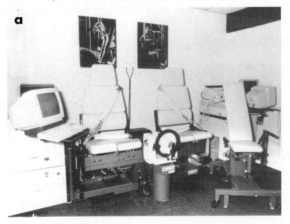

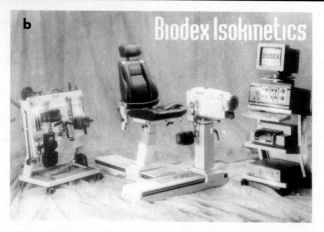

Figure 1-1 Two common isokinetic dynamometers currently on the market. a) the Cybex 6000; b) the Biodex (Courtesy of Biodex Medical Systems Inc.).

B. Muscle strength: terms and definitions

Several biomechanical factors influence the magnitude of force development, and these are explained below (Harman 1994).

(a) Neural contraction: the type and number of motor units involved in a muscle contraction, and the rate of motor unit firing;

(b) Muscle cross-sectional area;

(c) Muscle fiber arrangement;

(d) Muscle length: as less force can be generated when the muscle is shorter or longer than its resting length (fewer cross-bridge sites are available between actin and myosin filaments);

(e) Joint angle: as the muscle length and force relationship and the geometric arrangement of muscles, tendons and joint structures influence subsequent torque production;

(f) Muscle contraction velocity;

(g) Strength-to-Mass ratio reflects the ability to accelerate one's body;

(h) Body size: the smaller athletes are in advantage as they have higher strength-to-mass ratio than large athletes.

1. Types of muscle action

There are three distinct types of muscle action. They are classified by the nature of the applied load or by the velocity and direction of change in the length of the muscle (Lieber 1992).

The three types of action are concentric (shortening), isometric (static) and eccentric (lengthening) (Figure 1-2). Concentric and eccentric actions are dynamic and are involved in both dynamic and isokinetic exercises, whereas an isometric action is static. Muscle tension generated is greatest in eccentric and least in concentric actions (Lieber 1992). The terms describing muscle actions have often been used interchangeably, with terms describing modes of muscle strength testing (Sapega 1990). It is important to distinguish between the two.

a. Concentric action

In concentric muscle actions, the distance between the origin and the insertion of the muscle becomes shorter as it develops tension. The force developed depends on the muscle tension required to move the load, which varies with joint position (Figure 1-2a).

b. Isometric action

In isometric, or static, actions, the muscle acts to develop tension against an immovable object or resistance. The distance between the origin and the insertion does not change, and no movement of the lever arm occurs. Although there is no overall shortening of the muscle, there will be some shortening of the sarcomeres and some stretching of elastic structures in series with those sarcomeres, such as tendons and connective tissue. The development of tension during isometric action depends on the degree of voluntary effort exerted by the subject (Figure 1-2b).

c. Eccentric action

In eccentric actions, the muscle is forced to lengthen while contracting, and the distance between the origin and the insertion increases. The muscular force developed is overcome by an opposing external force, and the muscle merely provides active resistance as the opposing force stretches it to a more lengthened position (Figure 1-2c). Eccentric actions generate greater muscular tension and require less muscle work than concentric actions (Lieber 1992). Eccentric training can be associated with delayed onset of muscle soreness (DOMS) (Jones and Rutherford 1987), possibly due to mechanical and biochemical causes. The former involves tissue swelling followed by disruption of the extracellular matrix as a result of muscle injury, producing pain and inflammation. Biochemical mechanisms involve the release of histamine, kinins and prostaglandins in response to tissue damage, leading to pain (MacIntyre et al 1995).

Human movements rarely involve pure forms of isolated concentric, eccentric or isometric actions. Many running and jumping activities involve eccentric and concentric components, one following immediately after the other, sometimes preceded by an isometric action, as in a sprint start. The combination of eccentric and concentric action forms a natural type of muscle function, known as stretch-shortening cycle (SSC) (Komi 1984, Norman and Komi 1979). This SSC is used in plyometric training, especially by athletes involved in activities which require jumping and running.

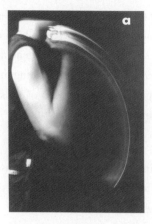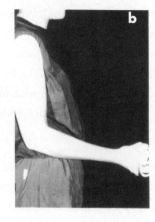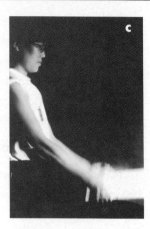

Figure 1-2 Different modes of muscle action. a) concentric; b) isometric; c) eccentric action.

2. Muscle strength and related terms

a. Strength

The term muscle strength refers to the capacity of a muscle to actively develop tension, irrespective of the specific conditions under which this is measured. Almost all modes of expression of muscular strength are directly related to each other. Clinical tests which measure strength evaluate the capacity of a subject's given muscle group to develop maximum voluntary tension. The units of measurement are linear or rotational force. Although the appropriate word for their rotational force is moment, the term torque has been widely used, and will be used in this text. Torque is measured in Newton meters.

b. Work

Work is defined as the output of mechanical energy, or externally applied force multiplied by the distance through which it is applied (force x distance and, in isokinetics, rotation). It is a useful measure of energy expenditure, and it is expressed in joules (J).

c. Power

Power refers to the rate of muscular work output. It is expressed in units of work per unit of time (Joules/second)/(Watts).

d. Endurance

Endurance is the ability of muscles to perform repeated contractions against a load for a prolonged period.

e. Explosive power

Explosive power refers to the time taken to reach peak power.

C. Modes of testing muscle strength

1. Isometric mode

The isometric mode of muscle strength testing involves contraction against a fixed, immovable object. Strength is measured as the peak force or torque developed during a maximal voluntary contraction. A high degree of accuracy is possible with various tensiometers. Test-re-test reliability is typically high (Sapega 1990). As most sports movements are dynamic rather than static, the isometric method, though relatively popular, may not be ideal in the routine assessment of muscle characteristics of athletes.

2. Isoinertial or dynamic variable-resistance mode

Isoinertial testing involves variable speed of movement with fixed resistance, such as the use of free weights or machines. Isoinertial exercises are composed of concentric and eccentric actions and are commonly known as "isotonic". The term "isoinertial", however, is more scientifically correct, and should be used instead (Abernethy et al 1995). Normally, the term isotonic is considered synonymous with concentric. Isoinertial strength is measured as the heaviest weight which can be lifted once through a given ROM. The reliability of isoinertial testing is generally good, although difficulty in controlling inertial forces that develop with differing lifting techniques makes weightlifting somewhat imprecise when applied to the study of muscular performance in humans (Sapega 1990). This method is not often used for scientific purposes.

3. Isokinetic mode

Isokinetic exercise is defined as dynamic muscular contraction when velocity of movement is controlled and held constant by a special isokinetic device (Thistle et al 1967). The resistance of the device equals the applied muscular torque throughout the ROM. This is, however, not true at the beginning and at the end of a given motion. Therefore, isokinetic movements require the use of an electromechanical appliance capable of maintaining a constant velocity of movement. Muscle contractions are not themselves isokinetic: concentric and eccentric contractions may be produced by isokinetic exercises, depending on the testing modes of a given apparatus. Table 1-1 describes some of the main advantages and disadvantages associated with isometric, isoinertial and isokinetic modes of muscle testing. The choice of testing modality depends on the objectives of the assessment, and on availability of equipment, time and personnel.

	Advantages	Disadvantages
Isometric	*useful if joint movement is painful or contraindicated *minimal equipment required *easy to perform *convenient for bed or home exercise *no cost	*lack of dynamic functions *strength increase in joint is largely angle-specific *little objective feedback of strength increases
Isoinertial	*progression is obvious *includes concentric and eccentric modes *minimal equipment needed *allows exercise of multiple joints *convenient for home exercises	*maximal loading occurs at the weakest point in ROM *momentum factor involved once the weight starts moving *stronger muscle groups can compensate for weaker ones during lifting of free weights *can be unsafe on already injured joints
Isokinetics	*maximal dynamic loading through muscles ROM *objective, reproducible and quantifiable assessment *provides speed-specific training through the velocity in a given range *isolation of weak muscle groups by strapping and limiting ROM to a specific angle of movement *accommodating resistance provides additional safety *good for early muscle rehabilitation *functional pattern training possible	*time consuming *requires specially trained personnel *cost of equipment

Table 1-1 Advantages and disadvantages of the three modes of muscle testings.

II. Available Technology, Reliability and Variables of Interest

A. Commonly used isokinetic dynamometers

Table 2-1 describes some of the facilities, functions and specifications provided by four commonly used isokinetic dynamometers on the market.

	Cybex	Kin-Com	Biodex	Lido
Common models on the market	II+, 340, 350, 6000	500H, 125e+, AP	2000	Active MJ
Most updated models	6000	AP	2000	Active MJ
Modes available	Ecc, Con, CPM	Con, Ecc, CPM	Con,Ecc, Isometric	Con, Ecc, CPM
Speed spectrum	0°-450°Con 0°-120°Ecc	1°-250°		1°-400°Con 1°-250°Ecc 1°-180°CPM
Specifications	*Double knee chair *Gravity elimination *Data base *Progress & fatique data comparison *Trunk muscles application	*Single & double chair *Trunk muscle application *Gravity elimination *Progress & fatigue data comparison *Measures force at source	*Single chair *Trunk muscle application *Progress & fatigue data comparison	*Single chair *Gravity elimination *Upgradable *Normative database software

Con = concentric, Ecc = eccentric, CPM = continuous passive motion

Table 2-1 Commonly used isokinetic models.

B. Function of isokinetics

Isokinetic techniques are currently used for five major purposes: strength testing, rehabilitation, research, diagnosis of injury, and, to some extent, as a training aid.

1. Evaluation

The main function of isokinetics probably lies in evaluation of muscle strength as it provides a wide range of information on dynamic performance variables of a muscle group, such as torque, work, explosiveness and endurance (Kannus 1994). Many feel that isokinetics can offer a greater degree of objectivity than other methods (Urquhart et al 1995). This is mainly because the calculation of force, work and power is difficult in other forms of dynamic exercise, where velocity is not controlled and because the changing mechanical advantage, as in weightlifting of the limb-lever system alters the force applied to the muscles through the ROM (Laird and Rozier 1979). Isokinetic testing has been successfully employed in the measurement of strength in patients with sports injuries (Yeung et al 1994), with various neuromuscular conditions (Watkins et al 1984), and in screening athletes (Morrissey et al 1995).

2. Rehabilitation

The variable resistance offered by isokinetic machines provides safety when treating musculo-tendinous injuries (Baltzopoulos and Brodie 1989, Stanton and Purdam 1989, Timm 1988). This is one of the major advantages they offer. Especially in early rehabilitation, patients are often unable to exercise at slower velocities which require the development of maximum tension (Perrin 1993). The velocity of isokinetic exercises can be modified to suit the capabilities of the patient. Muscle force varies at different joint angles (Huijing 1992), and the major advantage of isokinetic exercise is that the resistance of the dynamometer is proportional to the muscles capacity at all angles. Pain and muscle fatigue are constantly accommodated and a greater degree of safety and effectiveness is achieved (Osternig 1986). An additional advantage, especially in injury assessment and rehabilitation, is that no return movement of the limb-lever arm is required, thus avoiding potentially damaging eccentric contractions, inherent in all gravity-loaded systems (MacIntyre et al 1995). Many isokinetic dynamometers have a continuous passive motion (CPM) facility, which allows early mobilization of a given joint without the associated joint forces which occur with muscle contractions (Perrin 1993). All these features combine to permit early commencement of rehabilitation, especially after surgery.

3. Research work

As isokinetic dynamometry offers the possibility of quantifiable assessment of dynamic muscle function, providing information on a range of muscle characteristics, it has become a valuable tool for research work. Provided the test protocol is strictly adhered to, objective and accurate data on a wide range of variables can be generated (Perrin 1993) (Figure 2-1). Because isokinetic science is of interest to those within both Sports Medicine and Sports Science, the area of research has ranged from attempts to predict the likelihood of injuries in sport by assessing bilateral or ipsilateral muscle strength differences (Jonhagen et al 1994, Knapik et al 1991) to assessing the efficacy of various methods of strength training to functional performance in sport (Smith and Melton 1981). In the past 25 years, a considerable body of research has emerged, yet despite this a host of fundamental questions remains unanswered.

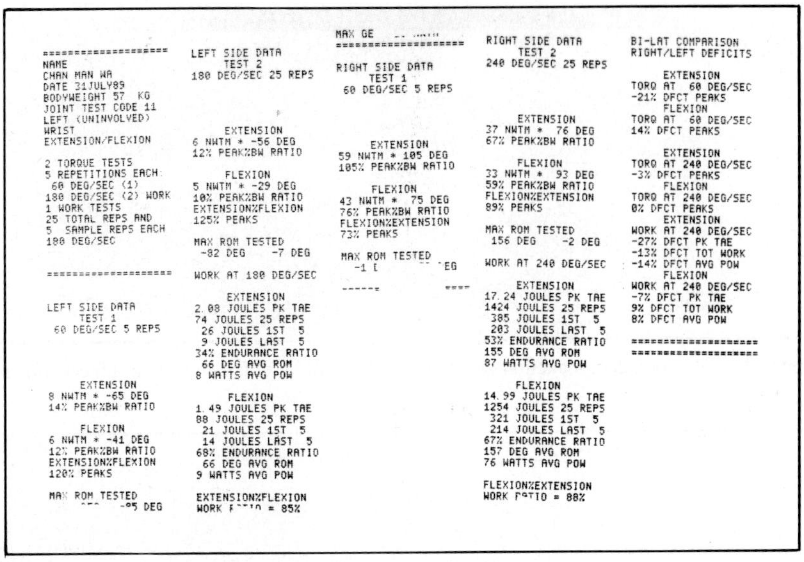

```
====================
NAME
CHAN MAN WA
DATE 31JULY89
BODYWEIGHT 57  KG
JOINT TEST CODE 11
LEFT (UNINVOLVED)
WRIST
EXTENSION/FLEXION

2 TORQUE TESTS
5 REPETITIONS EACH:
 60 DEG/SEC (1)
180 DEG/SEC (2) WORK
1 WORK TESTS
25 TOTAL REPS AND
5  SAMPLE REPS EACH
180 DEG/SEC

====================

LEFT SIDE DATA
     TEST 1
 60 DEG/SEC 5 REPS

     EXTENSION
8 NWTM * -65 DEG
14% PEAK%BW RATIO

     FLEXION
6 NWTM * -41 DEG
12% PEAK%BW RATIO
EXTENSION%FLEXION
120% PEAKS

MAX ROM TESTED
            -95 DEG

LEFT SIDE DATA
     TEST 2
180 DEG/SEC 25 REPS

     EXTENSION
6 NWTM * -56 DEG
12% PEAK%BW RATIO

     FLEXION
5 NWTM * -29 DEG
10% PEAK%BW RATIO
EXTENSION%FLEXION
125% PEAKS

MAX ROM TESTED
 -82 DEG     -7 DEG

WORK AT 180 DEG/SEC

     EXTENSION
2.08 JOULES PK TAE
74 JOULES 25 REPS
 26 JOULES 1ST  5
 9 JOULES LAST  5
34% ENDURANCE RATIO
 66 DEG AVG ROM
8 WATTS AVG POW

     FLEXION
1.49 JOULES PK TAE
88 JOULES 25 REPS
 21 JOULES 1ST  5
 14 JOULES LAST  5
68% ENDURANCE RATIO
 66 DEG AVG ROM
9 WATTS AVG POW

EXTENSION%FLEXION
WORK RATIO = 85%

MAX GE
====================

RIGHT SIDE DATA
     TEST 1
 60 DEG/SEC 5 REPS

     EXTENSION
59 NWTM * 105 DEG
105% PEAK%BW RATIO

     FLEXION
43 NWTM *  75 DEG
76% PEAK%BW RATIO
FLEXION%EXTENSION
73% PEAKS

MAX ROM TESTED
  -1 [           EG

------          ----

RIGHT SIDE DATA
     TEST 2
240 DEG/SEC 25 REPS

     EXTENSION
37 NWTM *  76 DEG
67% PEAK%BW RATIO

     FLEXION
33 NWTM *  93 DEG
59% PEAK%BW RATIO
FLEXION%EXTENSION
89% PEAKS

MAX ROM TESTED
 156 DEG     -2 DEG

WORK AT 240 DEG/SEC

     EXTENSION
17.24 JOULES PK TAE
1424 JOULES 25 REPS
 385 JOULES 1ST  5
 203 JOULES LAST  5
53% ENDURANCE RATIO
155 DEG AVG ROM
87 WATTS AVG POW

     FLEXION
14.99 JOULES PK TAE
1254 JOULES 25 REPS
 321 JOULES 1ST  5
 214 JOULES LAST  5
67% ENDURANCE RATIO
157 DEG AVG ROM
76 WATTS AVG POW

FLEXION%EXTENSION
WORK RATIO = 88%

BI-LAT COMPARISON
RIGHT/LEFT DEFICITS

      EXTENSION
TORQ AT  60 DEG/SEC
-21% DFCT PEAKS
      FLEXION
TORQ AT  60 DEG/SEC
14% DFCT PEAKS

      EXTENSION
TORQ AT 240 DEG/SEC
-3% DFCT PEAKS
      FLEXION
TORQ AT 240 DEG/SEC
0% DFCT PEAKS
      EXTENSION
WORK AT 240 DEG/SEC
-27% DFCT PK TAE
-13% DFCT TOT WORK
-14% DFCT AVG POW
      FLEXION
WORK AT 240 DEG/SEC
-7% DFCT PK TAE
9% DFCT TOT WORK
8% DFCT AVG POW

====================
====================
```

Figure 2-1 A data report of a wrist test using Cybex II+ isokinetic dynamometer.

4. Diagnosis

Isokinetics can be used as an adjunct in the diagnosis of injuries. As a joint moves through its ROM, objective information can be gained from deviation from normal in the torque curve (Urquhart et al 1995). For example, anterior knee pain tends to result in a torque curve which is dramatically flattened with a drastically wavy plateau occurring through the mid-ROM. Such a curve is mainly caused by pain, leading to a corresponding drop in force output. Although this seems easy and convenient, it is essential to remember that a diagnostic curve is not always evident despite a definite pathology, and, conversely, abnormalities in the curve may be present in the absence of a real abnormality (Figures 2-2, 2-3, 2-4).

5. Training aid

An additional function of isokinetics lies in athletic training. Isokinetic techniques allow training at different and controlled speeds, which may make it more relevant to specific sports applications (Morrissey et al 1995). Research findings on the effectiveness of isokinetic training in improving sports performance are contradictory. High costs has so far limited the development of sport-specific training protocols.

C. Facilities offered

1. Measurement of force or torque

Isokinetic dynamometers measure angular velocity, the position of the moving body part,

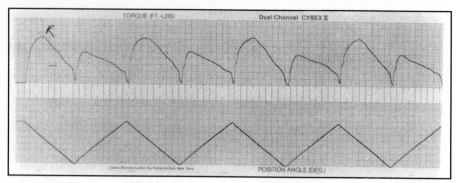

Figure 2-2 A Cybex data reduction computer (CDRC) curve obtained from a subject with an uninjured knee.

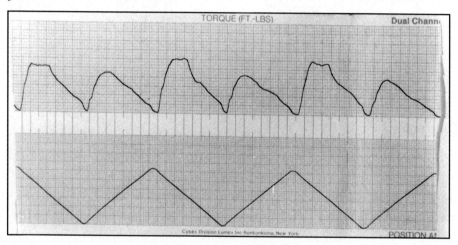

Figure 2-3 A CDRC curve obtained from a patient with anterior knee pain.

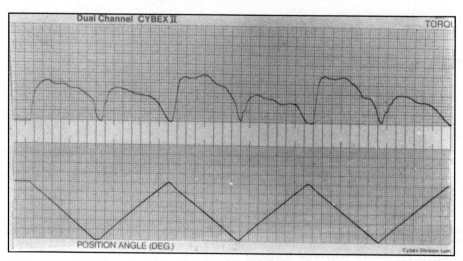

Figure 2-4 A CDRC curve obtained from a subject with an uninjured knee exhibiting a specific abnormalities.

and either force or torque. If the force-sensing apparatus, (the load cell), is located in the axis of rotation, the instrument measures torque. Force measurements are made when the load cell is situated distally on the resistance lever arm, as in the Kin-Com isokinetic dynamometer. Torque measurements can be calculated from here if necessary.

2. Control of speed

The mechanism controlling the speed systems in most common dynamometers consists of either an electronic servo-motor or a hydraulic valve which theoretically prevents acceleration of the limb irrespective of increases in force applied once the preset speed has been attained. For example, control in the Kin-Com is accomplished through feedback loops which monitor the position and speed of the lever arm and the force exerted by the user. It uses a strain gauge bridge to measure force and a bar-encoded shaft for position and speed measurements. These dynamic devices function in such a way that a degree of initial acceleration and final deceleration tend to be unavoidable. Manufacturers have attempted to prevent, dampen, correct for or exclude such inertial artifacts, commonly known as "overshooting" (Sapega 1990). For example, the Cybex II+ recorder has a damping knob on the torque channel, which controls the speed of response of the torque stylus. This dampens out unwanted, high frequency oscillation although these adjustments are not often thought satisfactory. Newer models (eg, Cybex 6000) do this automatically.

3. Active - passive modes

Dynamometers are either active or passive. Passive dynamometers provide resistance only, and measure either concentric or isometric forces. Active dynamometers, such as the Kin-Com, the Cybex 6000 and Biodex are capable of producing eccentric action in addition to concentric and isometric actions at preset angular velocities. These dynamometers also allow CPM. CPM training can be an important modality during early mobilization following surgery.

4. Concentric and eccentric mode

All isokinetic dynamometers measure concentric muscle actions. Eccentric actions develop greater tension than concentric muscle actions made at the same angle, and may therefore be more effective in improving muscle strength (Albert 1995). Eccentric action produces greater loading of the elastic components, which may help to improve sprinting and jumping performance, and may be useful in the rehabilitation of, for example, Achilles tendinitis (Kellis and Baltzopoulos 1995). A functional need for the eccentric mode exists, as many dynamic movements, such as walking downhill, or the point of impact of the tennis backhand involves an eccentric component. Muscle tears tend to occur during eccentric muscle action and, if the ability of the muscle to resist forces was improved, the risk of strains and tears might be reduced (Bennett and Stauber 1986). On the other hand, the eccentric movements produced by isokinetic machines are considered by some to be "unnatural", as described earlier, and their training effect appears to be very specific (Kannus 1994). An eccentric action within a sporting movement is normally short and occurs through few degrees of movement, whereas isokinetic eccentric movement is performed through the full ROM.

5. Range of test velocities

It has been shown that during concentric isokinetic testing muscle, torque decreases with increasing angular velocity of movement. Figure 2-5 describes the force-velocity relationship. The ability of a muscle to generate concentric force is the greatest at slow isokinetic velocities and decreases linearly as the test velocity increases. The reverse happens during eccentric muscle actions. Eccentric force remains the same, or increases with increasing test velocity. The difference between the force-velocity relationship during eccentric and concentric actions are attributed to differences in the binding and interaction of actin and myosin within the muscle sarcomere (for a more detailed discussion, see Albert 1995, MacIntyre et al 1995, Baltzopoulos and Brodie 1989). However, this does not hold true for many athletes, who have gained specific neuromuscular adaptations from event-specific training. Normally, two or three speeds are required in testing, including slow (30°/s to 60°/s), medium (90°/s to 120°/s) and fast (180°/s to 300°/s) speed. Table 2-2 illustrates the speeds commonly used for testing of the knee, shoulder, ankle and trunk muscles. The hip and the wrist have been excluded because of the difficulties associated with the testing of such respectively large and small movements with many of the dynamometers currently available. The fast speeds used for testing athletes are normally greater than those used for "normal" subjects and patients.

Because of the phenomenon of physiological strength overflows, improvements may be produced in speeds above and below the training speed itself (Timm 1987). Although conclu-

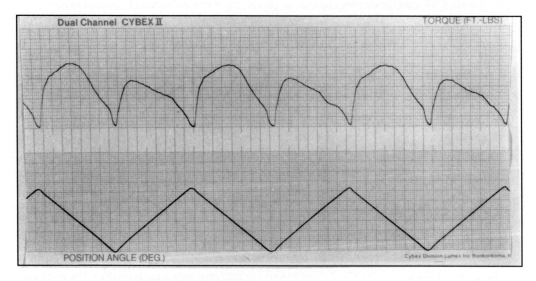

Figure 2-5 Concentric and eccentric force-velocity curve.

	Slow	Medium	High (Patients)	High(Athletes)
Knee Con	60	120	180	240-300
Knee Ecc	30	-	120	120
Shoulder Con	60	120	180	240
Shoulder Ecc (flex/ext)	30	-	120	120
Ankle Con	60	120	180	180-240
Ankle Ecc	-	-	-	-
Trunk Con	30	90	120	120
Trunk Ecc	-	-	-	-

Note: Testing modes Con= concentric; Ecc= eccentric.
Speeds are expressed in degrees per second (°/s).

Table 2-2 Velocities used in the Hong Kong Sports Institute (HKSI) in testing the knee, ankle, shoulder and the trunk.

sive evidence is lacking, velocity spectrum training is often advocated to stimulate both slow and fast muscle fibers. Specificity of speed is particularly important in athletic training (Moffroid and Whipple 1990). Some feel, however, that in isokinetic exercise, velocity spectrum training is not necessary, because isokinetic exercise provides maximum resistance at all speeds, and both slow and fast fibers will be recruited at slower velocities (Perrin 1993). In practice, even the fastest isokinetic velocities do not approach the angular joint velocities recorded in actual sporting situations. The same applies to all other modes of resistance training. Patients undergoing rehabilitation and unable to tolerate the higher levels of tension required in slow isokinetic exercise are often able to train at higher velocities because this tends to load the joint less. This is particularly true at the early stages of rehabilitation. However, fast eccentric isokinetic training has been associated with the possibility of soft-tissue injury (Perrin 1993). In practice, the velocities required of an isokinetic machine range between zero and 360°/s.

Practical Example

As a practical example, try to move the arm up and down (180° each time) ten times as fast as possible. Check how long it takes to complete the task. This ought to demonstrate that 360°/s is a fast speed and difficult to perform with added resistance.

---

6. Minimum and maximum force or torque limits

Dynamometers are limited in the accommodating resistance they can provide for safety reasons, and currently torque limits range from 250 foot-pounds (ft-lb) (Cybex 6000, CPM mode) to 500 ft-lb (Cybex and Merac). The lower levels are appropriate for testing the upper body segments, while higher levels are required for the trunk, hips and thighs (Perrin 1993). Elite athletes will often exceed these limits, especially when using the eccentric mode and when testing the powerful action of the hip. Indeed, manufacturers of certain isokinetic equipment have issued special instructions for the testing of the hip because of potential damage to the machine. Damage is possible in machines, such as Cybex which does not measure force at source.

7. Gravity control

In many test positions, for example, knee extension and flexion in the sagittal plane (gravity acting plane), only gravity will either aid or oppose the movement and thus influence the torques produced (Thorstensson et al 1976). Large errors may be recorded in mechanical work, up to 510% in knee extension (Winter et al 1981), if gravity is not accounted for. The Cybex, for instance, uses a data reduction computer (CDRC) to automatically adjust its calculations to incorporate the weight of the limb being tested. Gravity correction is not required for the measurement of shoulder internal/external rotation, ankle and trunk movements. An example of a gravity corrected CDRC graph of a normal knee can be seen in Figure 2-6.

8. Pre-loading and performance

Isometric studies have shown that the time to reach maximum tension from the onset of muscle activity on the EMG will take 250ms or more (Gransberg and Knuttson1983). In isokinetic knee extension at 240°/s, with unloaded acceleration, peak force will occur at approximately 200ms from the onset of contraction. Therefore, peak force will be recorded before

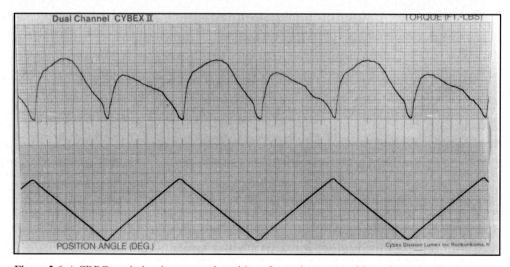

Figure 2-6 A CDRC graph showing a normal quadriceps/hamstrings curve with gravity correction.

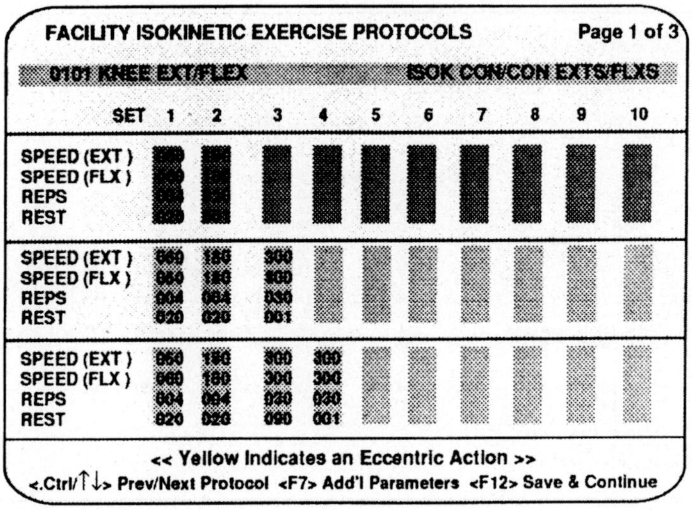

Figure 2-7 A typical protocol matrix — a sample of the facility of isokinetic exercise protocols provided by the Cybex 6000 dynamometer.

maximum tension could have been reached. A pre-load or a start force is used to prevent movement from starting before a certain force has been achieved (Gransberg and Knuttson1983). This eliminates the problem of variation in the time needed to reach maximum tension. Some devices have static (eg, Kin-Com and Cybex 6000) and some have dynamic pre-loading systems. Static pre-loading requires the operator-selected force to be applied on the given limb before motion is allowed. Dynamic pre-loading refers to passive loading of the given muscle group by stretching it immediately before the contraction starts (Jensen et al 1991). Static pre-loading provides a more accurate measurement of maximal dynamic muscle performance at the beginning of movement (Gransberg and Knuttson 1983).

9. Test and exercise protocols built into the machine software

A menu of protocols for testing or exercising different joints in a wide variety of patterns is offered by modern isokinetic dynamometers. Clinicians tend to create their own protocols suited for the particular needs and capabilities of their individual patients. For rehabilitation, it is possible to run different protocols in sequence, linking together a number of exercises. Figure 2-7 illustrates the facility protocol of the Cybex 6000.

10. Data output facility of the software

This is particularly important for those who wish to use isokinetic equipment for research purposes. Some software is designed to provide convenient data collection and storage, and is particularly suited for research. In the 1970s, data output consisted of the torque graph and all the calculations had to be based on this. Most modern machines give data on torque, power, work and range of movement against time and at different velocities. It is also possible to obtain

```
FACILITY    : Prince of Wales Hospital          CYBEX EVALUATION     PG 1 OF 1
CLIENT NAME: Guo, Xia                           CLIENT ID      : P419180
REPORT DATE: 07/03/1995   18:24                 REPORT TYPE    : ISKD BILATERAL
MUSCLE GRP : EXTERNAL ROTATORS                  CURR BW (kgs):  61
DAP/ACTION : 0109 SHOULDER INTERNAL/EXTERNAL ROTATION CON/ECC

SIDE(S) TESTED / DATE :   L   07/03/1995    R   07/03/1995   DEFICIT
BW (kgs) / MAX GET (Nm):   61      0          61      0
REPS                        5      5           5      5

                   CONCENTRIC EXTERNAL ROTATORS
SPEED(S) (deg/sec)         60     120          60     120        60    120
PEAK TORQUE (Nm)           14      9           11      8         22%   12%
PEAK TORQUE % BW           22%    14%          18%    13%
ANGLE OF PEAK TORQUE       24     17           20     14
TORQUE @ -30 deg            9      7            5      5         45%   29%
TORQUE @  30 deg           14      9           11      8         22%   12%
ACCEL TIME (sec)
TOTAL WORK (BWR) (J)       20     14           14     12         30%   15%
TOTAL WORK (BWR) % BW      32%    22%          22%    19%
AVG POWER (BWR) (watts)    10     11            6      9         40%   19%
AVG POWER (BWR) % BW       16%    18%           9%    14%
TAE (J)
ASD (Nm)                    1      0            0      0
SET TOTAL WORK (J)         85     64           52     53         39%   18%
ENDURANCE RATIO
50% FATIGUE WORK (J)
50% FATIGUE TIME (sec)
50% FATIGUE REPS
WORK RECOVERY RATIO
```

Figure 2-8 A data report providing information of bilateral discrepancy under "deficit" column.

```
FACILITY    : Prince of Wales Hospital          CYBEX EVALUATION     PG 1 OF 2
CLIENT NAME: Cheng, chi wa                      CLIENT ID      : K0111880
REPORT DATE: 07/04/1995   13:22                 REPORT TYPE    : ISKD PROGRESS
MUSCLE GRP : EXTERNAL ROTATORS                  CURR BW (kgs):  77
DAP/ACTION : 0109 SHOULDER INTERNAL/EXTERNAL ROTATION CON/ECC

SIDE(S) TESTED / DATE :   L   06/08/1995    L   06/15/1995   PROGRESS
BW (kgs) / MAX GET (Nm):   77      0          77      0
REPS                        5      5           5      5

                   CONCENTRIC EXTERNAL ROTATORS
SPEED(S) (deg/sec)         60     120          60     120        60    120
PEAK TORQUE (Nm)           22     16           22     18         0%    12%
PEAK TORQUE % BW           28%    20%          28%    23%
ANGLE OF PEAK TORQUE      -30      6           24     19
TORQUE @ -30 deg           22     14           16     15        -27%    7%
TORQUE @  50 deg           15      8           18     14         20%   75%
ACCEL TIME (sec)
TOTAL WORK (BWR) (J)       30     20           28     26         -6%   30%
TOTAL WORK (BWR) % BW      38%    25%          36%    33%
AVG POWER (BWR) (watts)    16     21           16     27         0%    28%
AVG POWER (BWR) % BW       20%    27%          20%    35%
TAE (J)
ASD (Nm)                    1      0            0      1
SET TOTAL WORK (J)        142     89          142    113         0%    28%
ENDURANCE RATIO
50% FATIGUE WORK (J)
50% FATIGUE TIME (sec)
50% FATIGUE REPS
WORK RECOVERY RATIO
```

Figure 2-10 A data report providing information of progress from the previous test unde under the "progress" column. A negative (-)symbol denotes a regression of a progression.

information at various points on the torque curve. Graphical data display can provide information on curve shape which can aid in the diagnosis of injury. The information provided allows assessment of dynamic muscle characteristics in terms of agonist/antagonist ratios, fatigue ratio, bilateral differences, and day-to-day progressive comparisons, as illustrated in Figures 2-8, 2-9. Please refer to "C. Facilities offered" in this Section for further information regarding variables which might be measured with isometric dynamometers. Modern software makes isokinetics subject-friendly in that immediate feedback can be given on performance and progression.

11. Limb and trunk measurement possibilities

One advantage of isokinetic machines is that for all the major joints it is possible to isolate and test movement in different planes, for example internal and external rotation of the shoulder, and plantar and dorsiflexions of the ankle. It is also possible to provide PNF pattern movements (Figure 2-10).

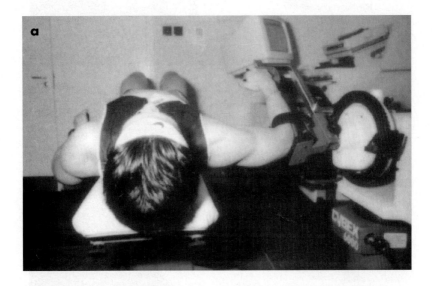

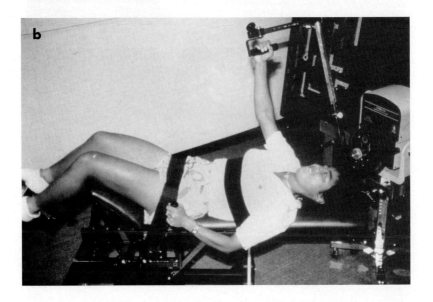

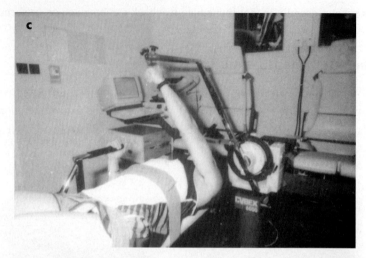

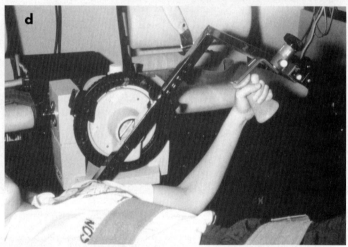

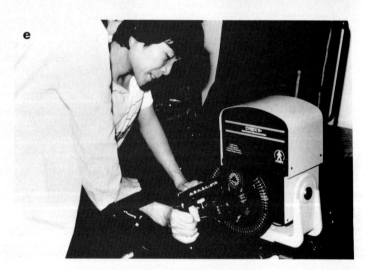

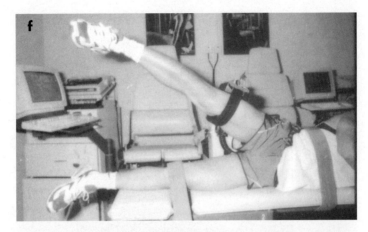

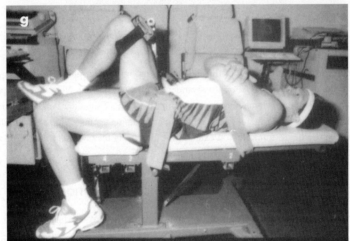

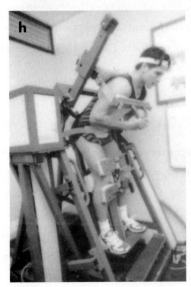

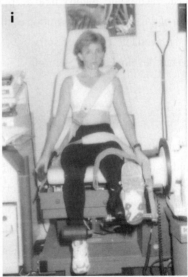

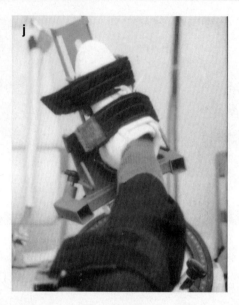

Figure 2-10 Examples of isokinetic testing of different joints and movement planes. a) shoulder internal/external rotation testing with shoulder at 90° abduction; b) shoulder PNF pattern testing. Note that the upper body exercise table (UBXT) is at an angle with the dynamometer to obtain the effect; c) shoulder horizontal abduction/adduction testing; d) elbow flexion/extension testing; e) wrist radial/ulnar deviation testing; f) hip abduction/adduction testing; g) hip flexion/extension testing; h) trunk flexion/extension testing using the Cybex TEF unit; i) knee flexion/extension testing; j) ankle inversion/eversion testing.

12. Comparability of data from different isokinetic machines

The literature suggests that despite the basic similarities of different devices, data obtained from isokinetic machines are not comparable, even if tests have been done in an identical manner. Extrinsic factors are mainly held responsible, including differences in positioning and stabilization of the subject, configuration of the instrument, and manipulation of the raw data on torque by the available computer software (Sapega 1990). Especially the Chattanooga group (Kin-Com) has developed new methods of joint stabilization.

D. Reliability of isokinetic dynamometry

The reliability of specific isometric dynamometers has generally been reported to be high. Several studies have tested the reliability and validity of isokinetic instrumentation in measuring torque, work and power (Magnusson et al 1990, Montgomery et al 1989, Bemben et al 1988, Farrell and Richards 1986, Mawdsley and Knapik 1982, Molnar and Alexander 1977, Moffroid et al 1969). All these studies indicate that the technical accuracy and reliability of isokinetics are very high, as correlation coefficients between the computed mechanical work value and measured work ranges between 0.93 and 0.99.

Although instrument reliability is high, attention and care must be exercised and a multitude of factors must be considered to ensure reproducible results when testing muscular performance.

1. Mechanical reliability

A trained technician is normally responsible for the maintenance of isokinetic equipment. A simple test can be performed by hanging a sufficiently heavy weight on the load cell of the instrument and noting the time required to move through a known distance at a specific angular velocity. If, however, the moment is being calibrated then the calculated moment is examined against the recorded moment.

2. Influence of the tester on reliability

It is essential that in all occasions the same testing procedures are strictly adhered to, including subject familiarization, subject set-up, warm-up and testing protocol (Urquhart et al 1995, Kannus 1994, Osternig 1986). A description of the test protocols used for the major joints in the HKSI (which will be addressed as "our laboratory" in the followings) is detailed in Section 3.

3. Influence of the subject on reliability

This can be difficult to control, as ability to comply may be influenced by the discomfort and pain sometimes associated with maximum exercise testing. Unaccustomed modes of exercise may also influence the outcome. Novices tend to have more difficulties, particularly performing eccentric contractions, and especially at higher speeds. In most cases, reliability coefficients for eccentric peak torque values tend to fall below those of concentric peak torques (Perrin 1993).

4. Reliability of testing different body regions

An overview of reliability studies involving different isokinetic dynamometers and different joint movements is provided in Table 2-3. In general, motions of easily isolated joints, such as the knee, tend to provide better reliability coefficients than joints readily permitting involvement of accessory muscle groups, such as those around the elbow.

a. Shoulder

Certain shoulder movers, especially internal and external rotators, tend to show a greater reliability than extensors and flexors (Greenfield et al 1990, Perrin 1986). Test reliability is also related to the angle of testing. Shoulder extensors and flexors tested in a neutral position appear to give more reliable results, while the reliability decreases as 90° of abduction is approached (Choi 1995, personal communications). Trunk stability is important in preventing accesssory muscles involvement around the shoulder. However, Frisiello et al (1994) have highlighted that stabilization, and thus reliability, sometimes has to be compromised for the

Study (year)	No of Subjects	Sex	Mean age (years)	Machine/model	Joint	Movement	Modes	Variable measured	Speeds (°/s)	Repetitions	Interval between tests(days)	Statistic used	Reliability result
Li et al (1996)	46	M	25.5	Cybex 6000	knee	flex/ext	Con & Ecc	PT,TW, PW	60° 120°	5 25	7	ICC	0.78-0.93
Burnham et al (1995)	20	M	18.9	Cybex 340	shoulder	abd/add	Con	PT	0° & 60°	4	10	ICC	0.63-0.78
Frisiello et al (1994)	18	M & F	18.3	Biodex	shoulder	int rot / ext rot	Ecc	PT	90° 120°	3	7	ICC	0.75-0.83 / 0.78-0.86
Sleivert and Wenger (1994)	20+3	M+F	24.7	Cybex	ankle / knee	dorsiflexion/plantar-flexion / flex/ext	Con	PT	0° 120° 240° / 360° & 480°	3 sec 3	48 hours	ICC	0.55-0.76 / 0.64-0.94
Bandy and McLaughlin (1993)	10+10	M+F	23.0	Cybex 6000	knee	flex/ext	Con	PT / TW / PW	60° 180° 300°	3	7	ICC	0.94-0.97 / 0.88-0.98 / 0.81-0.96
Frontera et al (1993)	17 35	M F	60.2 60.0	Cybex II+	dominant elbow / dominant knee	flex/ext / flex/ext	Con	PT	60° 180° / 60° 240°	5 25 / 5 25	7-10	Pearson's CC (p<0.01) / Pearson's CC (p<0.01)	M-0.71-0.84 F-0.67-0.78 / M-0.68-0.77 F-0.58-0.74
Heitman and Kovaleski (1993)	12 (MR)	M	17.3	Lido Active	knee	flex/ext	Con	PT	90° 180° 300°	5	7	ICC	90°-->0.90 180°--0.64-0.83 300°--0.45-0.66
Kilfoil & St Pierre (1993)	4 4 (Polio)	M F	47.5 56.8	Cybex II+	knee	flex/ext	Con	PT / T 60° / T 45°	30° 60° 90° 180°	3	7	ICC	PT 0.81-0.99 / T 60° 0.89-0.99 / T 45° 0.87-0.99
Malerba et al (1993)	14 10	M F	17-58	Biodex	shoulder	int/ext rotation	Con / Ecc	PT	60° 120° 60°	3 Con 3 Ecc	7	ICC	0.60-0.95 0.44-0.92 0.81-0.93

Study	n	Sex	Age	Dynamometer	Joint	Movement	Contraction	Measure	Velocity/Angle	No.	Interval (days)	Reliability	Value
Steiner et al (1993)	6 / 13	M / F	Adult	Lido Active	knee	flex/ext	Ecc	PT, TW, PW	60° / 180°	3	5-11	ICC	0.58-0.96
Suomi et al (1993)	22 (MR)	M	30.3	Merac	knee / hip	ext / abd	Con	PT & PW	60° / 30°	10	1	ICC	0.97-0.99 / 0.98-0.99
Gleeson and Mercer (1992)	10 / 8	M / F	28.4 / 27.5	Lido 2.1	knee	flex/ext	Con	PT	60° / 180°	4	5	ICC	0.881-0.994
Jablonowsky et al (1992)	20	M	17-30	ACE	leg & arm	ext/flex	Con	torque	ext 100° flex 125°	3 x 3	2	Test & re-test reliability	0.44-0.91
Kues et al (1992)	10	M	26.0	Kin-Com #500-11	right knee	extensor	Con / Ecc / Iso-metric	PT	30°, 90°, 120° & 180° / as above / 0°/s at 40° & 60° of knee flex	6	>48 & <96 hours	ICC	0.89-0.98 / 0.87-0.97 / 0.90-0.94
McCleary and Andersen (1992)	26	M	19.5	Biodex 2000	knee	flex/ext	Con	PT	60°	6	3	ICC	extension 0.97 flexion 0.98
Snow and Blacklin (1992)	11	F	26.0	Kin-Com	knee	flex/ext	Con	PT	30° / 180°	4	7	ICC	0.79-0.88
Weir et al (1992)	9 / 4	M / F	22	Cybex II+	knee	ext	Con	torque	0°/s at 45° knee flex	12	2	ICC	0.96
Wessel et al (1992)	30	F / M	18-56	Kin-Com	trunk	flex	Con & Ecc	PT	30°, 60° & 90°	3 x 3	5-8	ICC	>0.85
Wilhite et al (1992)	4 / 14	M / F	24.9	Kin-Com	knee	extensor	Con & Ecc	PT	60° / 120° / 180°	4	7	ICC	0.76-0.95
Delitto et al (1991)	29 / 32	M / F	20-60	Lidoback	trunk	flex/ext	Con	PT	60° / 120° / 180°	10	7-21	ICC	0.78-0.88

Study	n	Sex	Age	Dynamometer	Joint	Movement	Contraction	Measure	Angle/Velocity	Reps	Interval	Statistic	Reliability
Durand et al (1991)	14 (MR), 10 (Nor)	M, M	38.0, 33.0	Kin-Com	knee	flex/ext	Con	PT	30°, 180°	3	intertrial 2 mins	ICC	MR-0.74-0.93, Nor-0.86-0.93
Levene et al (1991)	11+9	M+F	20-37	Cybex 340	knee	flex/ext	Con	Maximum Average PT	60°, 180°	3	2	two-way ANOVA / ICC	no significant diff was found (p<0.05) / 0.98-0.99
Molczyk et al (1991)	20	F	24.8	Cybex II+	knee	flex/ext	Con	PT / Endurance	0°, 60°, 180°, 300°, 240° / 30	3	separate days	ICC	0.83-0.95, 0.88-0.95, 0.78-0.93, 0.69-0.93, 0.86-0.89
Tripp and Harris (1991)	14, 6	M, F	40.4, 22.7	Lido Active	knee	flex/ext	Con	PT	60°, 120°	5	2-4	ICC	0.92-0.97
Bohannon (1990)	20	F	29.2	Cybex II	knee	ext	Isometric	PT	0°	2 for 4-5 second each	intratrial	ICC	0.932
Burnett et al (1990)	29	M	6-10	Cybex II+	hip	flex/ext / abd/add	Con	PT	30° / 90°	4	7-14	ICC	highest 0.84 / <0.6
Feiring et al (1990)	19	M & F	20-35	Biodex	knee	flex/ext	Con	PT, TW	60°, 180°, 240°, 300°	5	7	ICC	PT-0.82-0.98, TW-0.95-0.97
Greenfield et al (1990)	20	M+F	25.3	Merac	right shoulder	rotation	Con	torque at 45° shoulder abduction	60°	3r	7	ICC	0.87
Kramer (1990)	15+20	M+F	25.7	Kin-Com	knee (dominant)	flex/ext	Con / Ecc	PT	45° / 90°	3	<10	ICC	0.81-0.91 / 0.79-0.87
Pitetti (1990)	19 (MR)	M, F	12, 7	Cybex 340	dominant knee / dominant elbow	flex/ext / flex/ext	Con	PT, AP, BW	60°	3	2-4	CC	0.73-0.92 / 0.71-0.88
Thigpen et al (1990)	50	M, F	24.2, 24.6	Cybex (A) CDRC, Cybex (B) SCR	knee	flex/ext	Con	PT	60°, 240°	4	2	inter-machine reliability	0.982-0.998
Lagasse (1989)	26	M	22.1	Omnitron	knee	flex/ext	Con	PT	50mm/sec	3 reps	24 hours	ICC	0.94

Study	N	Sex	Age	Dynamometer	Joint	Movement	Mode	Variable	Speed/Angle	Reps	Interval	Reliability	Value
McCrory et al (1989)	19	M+F	19-32	Lido Active	knee	flex/ext	Con Ecc	PT	30°	4	2	ICC(R₁)	0.93-0.95 0.80-0.95
Montgomery et al (1989)	18 14	M F	27.0 28.5	electro-rebotic servo dynamometer	knee	flex/ext	Con	PT	10 speeds from 60° to 330°		2-4	CC	extension −.88 flexion −.79
Harding et al (1988)	14	F	21.6	Kin-Com	right knee	flex ext	Con	PT	60°	6 reps	different days	ICC	0.953 0.957
Wessel et al (1988)	5 13	M F	18-40	Kin-Com	knee	flex/ext	Con Ecc	Mean PT PT	60° 180°	6	7	ICC	Con−0.894 Ecc−0.845 Con−0.810 Ecc−0.827 Con−0.918 Ecc−0.854 Con−0.839 Ecc−0.914
Burdett et al (1987)	36	M+F		Cybex II	knee	extensor	Con	endurance	180° 240°	when PT of 1st rep ↓50%	>2	ICC	0.84 0.71
Griffin (1987)	20	F	26.6	Kin-Com	elbow	flex/ext	Con Ecc	PT	30° 120°	3 reps	30 minutes	ICC	0.72-0.83
Johnson and Seigel (1978)	40	F	17-50	Cybex II	knee	ext	Con	PT	180°	6r	1-5d	ICC	0.93-0.99

Where M=male, F= female, flex= flexor, ext= extensor, Con= Concentric mode of exercise, Ecc= Eccentric mode of exercise, PT= peak torque, PT= peak torque in Newton-meter (Nm), TW= total work output in joules, PW= power in watt, ICC= Interclass Correlation, CC= Correlation Coefficient, int/ext rot= internal/external rotators, MR= mentally retarded, Nor= normal subjects

We concluded that
1) More advanced models do not particularly show higher reliability;
2) Variables with greater numerical values (eg, Peak torque of the knee) show higher reliability than the lower numerical one (eg, PKTAE of the elbow);
3) Variables of concentric mode produce greater reliability than eccentric mode ones.

Table 2-3 Reliability of isokinetic dynamometry.

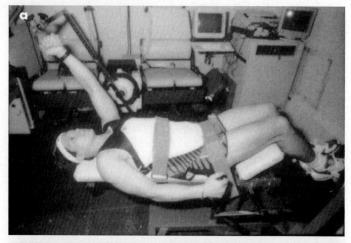

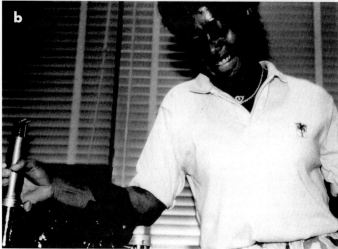

Figure 2-11 a) Shoulder flexion/extension testing. b) Shoulder internal/external rotation testing in neutral position.

safety of patient. Figure 2-11 shows the testing of shoulder flexion and extension, and internal and external rotation.

b. Knee

The reliability of quadriceps and hamstrings testing has been adequately established (Kannus 1994), and appears to be high across a variety of test speeds. The reliability of the eccentric mode again tends to be lower than the concentric mode (Kramer 1990, Klopfer and Greij 1988, Tredinnick and Duncan 1988, Burdett and VanSwearingen 1987).

c. Trunk

Published data on the reliability of trunk assessment are available only for the seated test position. Review of the literature reveals that the reliability of trunk extensor assessment tends to be good and consistent in normal subjects, regardless of test velocity (Friedlander et al 1995, Grabiner et al 1990, Smidt et al 1983). In patients with low back pain, the reliability of trunk flexion assessment improves with increased test velocity, as pain is associated with forceful muscle contractions related to low speed testing (Perrin 1993).

d. Ankle

Relatively few studies have considered the reliability of testing the ankle movements, and correlation coefficients for the concentric action vary from 0.67 to 0.94 (Cawthorn et al 1991, Wennerberg 1991, Karnofel et al 1989). Little reliability data exist for eccentric action.

e. Wrist and hip

The reliability of wrist and hip measurements tends to be low. The reason for this lack of reliability is associated with the large (hip) and small (wrist and ankle) ranges of movement typical of these joints. Lack of reliability is associated with the relatively small torque produced by the muscles in some joint movements. Any variation in the small torque value will therefore be magnified. Also, if the dynamometer does not register decimal points, greater variation in the results of a small movement test may occur.

Testing of the knee, ankle and trunk is shown in Figure 2-12.

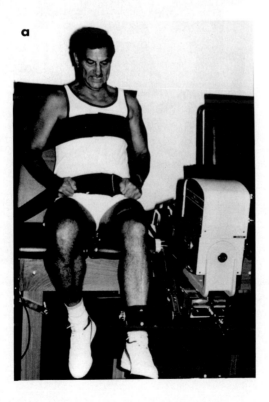

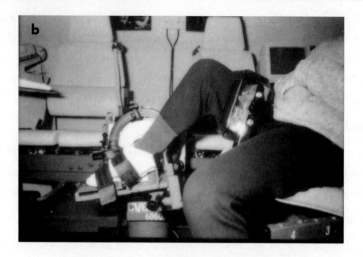

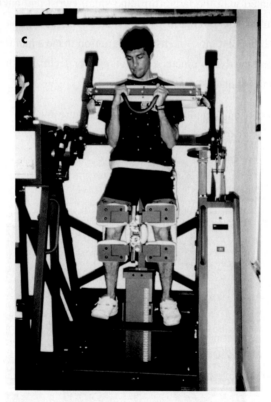

Figure 2-12 a) Knee flexion/extension testing. b) Ankle dorsiflexion/plantarflexion testing. c) Trunk flexion/extension testing using the Cybex TEF unit.

III. Scientific and Medical Aspects of Isokinetics

A. Isokinetics in Sports Medicine and Rehabilitation

1. Prevention of injuries

Many risk factors are associated with the occurrence of injury in sport (Requa et al 1993, Maffulli and Pintore 1990, Koplan et al 1985, Lysens et al 1984) (Figure 3-1). Their identification and study can be used for a systematic approach to prevention (Kannus 1993). Lack of muscle strength is considered to be one risk factor (Knapik et al 1991). Local muscle strength and that of surrounding structures, including tendons, ligaments and bone, together with some aspects of proprioception and motor control are all involved in injury prevention (Grimby 1992). Aspects of muscle strength which are sometimes evaluated for injury prevention include general muscle weakness, ipsilateral agonist/antagonist ratio, bilateral discrepancy, eccentric/concentric ratio, and endurance of a given muscle group. More recently, attention has been given to ipsilateral concentric agonist/eccentric antagonist work (Kellis and Baltzopoulos 1995). In general, the torque produced by a muscle or muscle group on opposite limbs is assumed to be fairly equal or "in balance". The ratio of the agonist and antagonist in the same extremity, for example hamstring and quadriceps, is also expected to be constant or "in balance", though not equal (Osternig 1986). A "physiological" range has been proposed (Kannus 1988), and it has been hypothesized that the weaker muscle group will be more susceptible to injury (Knapik et al 1991, Grace 1984). Muscle strength testing may therefore be used to prevent both primary and secondary injuries by screening for imbalances.

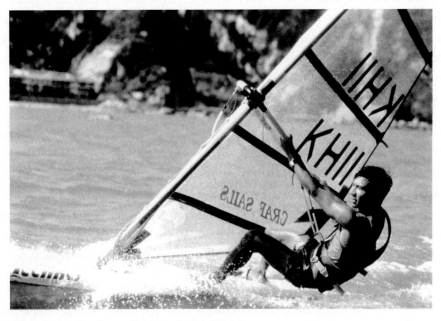

Figure 3-1 Windsurfing easily causes back injuries.

a. Muscle strength imbalance and injury

Muscle balance is the strength, power or endurance of one muscle or muscle group relative to another muscle or muscle group. Balance is often expressed in terms of relative strength between joint agonists and antagonists, or by contralateral comparisons. Muscles or muscle groups on opposite sides of a joint act reciprocally to produce smooth and coordinated movements. Therefore, deficiency in one muscle or muscle group may lead to an imbalanced action in that joint. Relatively few studies have investigated the relationship between imbalance in muscle strength and the occurrence of injuries. The issue is controversial, and stems from studies investigating previous joint injury and surgery leading to muscle weakness and imbalance, and a high rate of re-injury (Campbell and Wayne 1979, Marshall and Tischler 1978). More recently, Knapik et al (1991) investigated the relationship between pre-season strength and the incidence of injury in 138 female college athletes in a variety of weight-bearing sports. They reported that muscle imbalances measured at 180°/s were associated with injuries. Generally, those who support the hypothesis that muscle imbalance leads to injury argue that prophylactic selective strengthening programs may help to correct the weakness and the imbalance in uninjured joints, and thus reduce the rate of occurrence of injuries (Knight 1980, Slagle 1979, Cahill and Griffith 1978, Mulder 1973). Many studies have noted a large range of ratios in healthy populations. The prominence of strength training in post-operative rehabilitation has been universally emphasized (Kramer et al 1993, Kannus and Järvinen 1990). Most studies have focused on the knee joint because it is one of the largest and most complex joints in the body, which is frequently injured, frequently operated upon, and the impact of its impairment in the life of an athlete is significant. Also, return to normal function is vital if further injuries are to be prevented (Baltzopoulos and Brodie 1989). Certain areas of the body tend to be susceptible to injury. For example, the hamstrings in sprinters, jumpers and other power athletes, and the external rotators of the shoulders in swimmers, racket sports players and throwers may require specific training (Wathen 1994).

b. Agonist/antagonist ratios

The most commonly measured agonist/antagonist ratios include the knee extensions and flexions, shoulder internal and external rotation, shoulder abduction/adduction, shoulder flexion/extension, back flexion/extension, ankle plantarflexion/dorsiflexion, and ankle eversion/inversion. Isokinetic assessments of muscle imbalance are significantly influenced by a number of factors, including the test velocity, test angle, gravity, and the role of antagonist muscle coactivation. Effective use of isokinetic assessment is therefore dependent on a thorough understanding of the effects of these factors. Each will be now considered in turn.

Test velocity and the effect of gravity

Research on hamstring and quadriceps torque ratios (H:Q) has generally found that these values increase with increasing test speed. Osternig et al (1983) reported an increase in this ratio from 58% to 78% at speeds ranging from 50°/s to 400°/s. Schlinkman (1984) reported that the mean H:Q ratio in 342 collegiate football players increased from 54% at 60°/s to 67% at 300°/s. When the effect of gravity was taken into account, the ratio dropped by 8% to 12% when compared to non-gravity corrected values. At small joint angles, the gravitational torque is minimal and the error smaller, but, at large joint angles, it produces a larger error, and a decreased H:Q ratio (Baltzopoulos and Brodie 1989). Knee flexion/extension and hip abduction/adduction are easily affected by gravity, whereas movements of the wrist, ankle and shoulder internal/external rotation are not. It is now accepted that gravity corrected H:Q ratios do not increase with increasing test speeds (Kannus 1994).

Normally, peak torque (PT) tends to drop with increasing velocity. The drop in knee flexor torque has been found to be less than that in the knee extensors (Murray et al 1984, Osternig et al 1983). Consequently, at higher test speeds, hamstring torque moves closer to that of the quadriceps. Studies on H:Q strength ratio imbalance and the occurrence of injury have reported an association when muscle strength ratio was measured at 180°/s, but not at 30°/s (Knapik et al 1991). The proposed reason for this was that the higher speeds reflected more accurately the actual athletic activity of the subjects tested. Figure 3-2 shows a comparison of PT obtained using different angular velocities. In another study, we collected these data to illustrate the effect of angular velocity on force generation. Forty-two healthy males (aged 22.9±4.9 years) and 38 females (aged 21.2±2.8 years) were tested on the Cybex II+ dynamometer. Peak quadriceps and hamstrings torques of both limbs at angular velocities of 60°/s, 120°/s, 180°/s, 240°/s and 300°/s were determined. The mean peak torques dropped with each 60°/s increment.

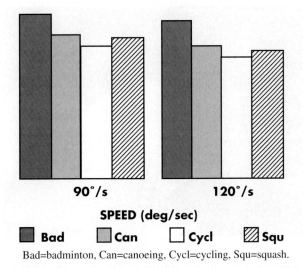

Bad=badminton, Can=canoeing, Cycl=cycling, Squ=squash.

Figure 3-2 The effect of speed on peak torque in four groups of athletes.

Angle of testing

Angular position is important in assessing muscle function because maximum torque production is dependent on optimal length of the muscle and thus on optimal joint angle. Figure 3-3 illustrates the effects of different angular positions in isokinetic testing. For example, Murray et al (1984) reported that, the H:Q ratio at 30° of knee flexion increased from 71% at 0°/s to 105% at 180°/s. At a joint angle of 60°, however, no major change was recorded with increasing speeds. This was explained as a reflection of rapidly falling force production in the quadriceps at higher speeds. The torque curve was also much flatter for the hamstring group throughout the ROM, and consequently there was less variability between two angles. Testing should approximate, as close as possible, the positional requirements of the sport or of the activity of daily living (Perrin 1993).

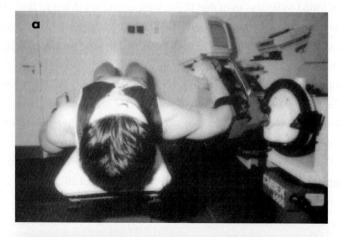

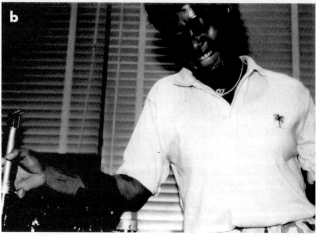

Figure 3-3 a) and b) Demonstrating the effect of different joint positions when testing the same movement — shoulder internal/external rotation.

Agonist/antagonist coactivation

Contraction of agonists may be associated with simultaneous contraction of their antagonists. Co-contraction of antagonists is common, particularly when the agonist contraction is strong and/or rapid, when the task requires precision, or when subjects are untrained in the task (Sale 1992). Co-contraction of antagonists may seem counterproductive, particularly when measuring muscle force production, as the opposing torque developed by the antagonists would decrease net torque in the intended direction of movement (Sale 1992). However, co-contraction has a protective role in maintaining joint stability and providing a braking mechanism, and may play a part in the coordination of the movement (Sale 1992). Toward the end of a single isokinetic movement, the limb decelerates as it approaches the limit of its articular excursion (Osternig et al 1983). In this respect, hamstring coactivation has been found to assist in the prevention of knee overextension during the swing phase of gait (Carlsoo et al 1973). Osternig et al (1985) investigated agonist/antagonist muscle coactivation in 9 intercollegiate track athletes performing maximal knee extensions and flexions at 100°/s and 400°/s. Simultaneously, integrated electromyographic (IEMG) activity was measured from quadriceps and hamstrings. They found that hamstring coactivation was considerably greater during knee extension than quadriceps coactivation during knee flexion. Hamstring coactivation was found to increase sharply during the last 25% of knee extension, and to be responsible for 58% of the IEMG agonist activity. Moreover, hamstring coactivation pattern was four times greater in sprinters than in distance runners. The authors suggested that the hamstrings are used to a much greater extent than the quadriceps for limb deceleration (eccentric activity), possibly because the powerful quadriceps group requires a greater degree of antagonist coactivation for deceleration. Antagonist EMG activity of the soleus has been reported to decrease with increasing velocity in isokinetic dorsiflexion (Nelson et al 1973) (Figure 3-4). In practice, co-contraction of antago-

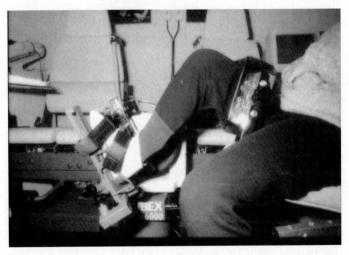

Figure 3-4 Ankle plantarflexion/dorsiflexion test.

nists may be either facilitated or inhibited depending on 1) external load of the agonist; 2) rhythmicity of the activity; and 3) velocity of limb movement (Osternig 1986). Agonist/antagonist coactivation introduces an error of estimation in torque values and may, consequently, distort the results of agonist/antagonist ratios.

(1) Agonist/antagonist ratio of the knee joint

Although the optimal values for agonist/antagonist ratios for the muscles around the knee joint are controversial, studies investigating the H:Q ratio suggest that this should be 50% to 80% depending on test velocity (Figure 3-5), although large inter-individual variation exists (Kannus 1988, Kannus and Järvinen 1990). Generally, a ratio of 60% measured at 60°/s is accepted as normal (Kellis and Baltzopoulos 1995). However, Nosse (1982) is skeptical of this value as it was derived isometrically, with flexors and extensors measured at a knee flexion angle of 15° and 65° respectively. Comparisons with other modes of testing are inaccurate because the length of the muscle and the mode of exercise are likely to influence the recorded ratio. Athletes engaged in, for example, rugby, which requires explosive push-offs and therefore a strong and powerful hamstring group, may require ratios closer to one. In injured knees, the long-term outcome appears to improve when the H:Q ratio approaches that of the uninjured limb (Kannus and Järvinen 1990). H:Q strength imbalance puts extra stress on the intra-articular ligaments of the knee. Consequently, the ability to restore the correct body alignment in response to sudden external forces is decreased. H:Q ratio imbalance in a cruciate deficient knee may alter joint kinematics, and thus decrease the functional capacity of the injured athlete. Interventional programs aimed at restoring the normal H:Q ratio while increasing quadriceps and hamstrings strength toward contralateral values support vigorous hamstring rehabilitation

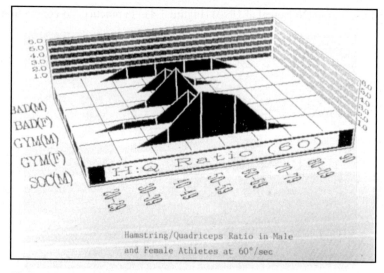

Hamstring/Quadriceps Ratio in Male
and Female Athletes at 60°/sec

Figure 3-5 H:Q ratio of different athletic groups measured at 60°/s falls mainly in the range of 50% to 60%.

(Li 1996).

(2) Agonist/antagonist ratios of the shoulder joint

Impingement syndrome is a common cause of shoulder pain and disability (Leroux et al 1994). Imbalance of the shoulder internal/external rotator ratio (SIR/SER) has been implicated as an etiological factor in impingement syndrome (Leroux et al 1994, Warner et al 1990, Jobe et al 1983). As the shoulder joint is a complex multiaxial joint capable of movement in multiple directions, valid and objective assessment of muscle function of this region is difficult. Moreover, variation in the testing position used in different studies makes interpretation and comparison of so-called "normative" data difficult (Perrin 1993). In general, the external rotator muscles generate torque of approximately 60% to 80% of the values generated by the internal rotator muscles. Corresponding values for the non-dominant side are slightly lower (Perrin 1993, Warner et al 1990). Factors affecting the SIR/SER ratio include sporting background. For example, McMaster et al (1991) reported a much lower ratio in water polo players, and Hinton (1988) in baseball pitchers. Shoulder flexion and extension occur through the sagittal plane. Isolation of the action of the shoulder flexors and extensors is difficult, because of the contribution of elbow flexors and extensors in maintaining elbow flexion (Perrin 1993). Normally, shoulder flexors are able to generate torque values of approximately 75% to 85% those recorded for the extensors (Pawlowski and Perrin 1989, Alderink and Kuck 1986, Berg et al 1985). In upper body sports, such as swimming and rowing, flexor muscles tend to produce only 50% of the force exerted by the extensors (Perrin 1993). In hitting the overhead smash in tennis, good eccentric strength is necessary to control external rotation of the shoulder and to prevent the shoulder joint from being dislocated, and damage the posterior nerves, leading to traction injury.

c. Bilateral discrepancy

A strength discrepancy of 10% to 15% or more between the two sides is considered to represent significant asymmetry (Elliot 1978, Gleim et al 1978). Such discrepancy is thought to predispose to injury at or around the given joint (Kannus 1994). Kannus (1994) has divided bilateral discrepancies into three subgroups (Table 3-1). Strength discrepancy of less than 10% is normal, 10% to 20% is possibly abnormal, and greater than 20% is probably abnormal. Achievement of 80% to 90% capability as measured in the uninvolved extremity is commonly

Bilateral strength discrepancy	
<10%	Normal
10-20%	Possibly abnormal
>20%	Probably abnormal

Table 3-1 The three subgroups of bilateral discrepancies (Kannus 1994).

used as a minimum standard for the involved extremity before the patient is allowed to return to sport after injury. Grace et al (1984) assessed the strength of knee flexors and extensors of 206 high school football players and correlated bilateral muscle strength differences with the occurrence of injury during the subsequent football season. They found no association between muscle imbalance of 10% or more and the frequency of injury, despite a high proportion of players with such an imbalance. So et al (1995) reported that significant bilateral differences can be expected in the shoulder joint of normal healthy young adults with no history of injuries to this region. Read and Bellamy (1990) studied strength ratios in tennis and squash players (asymmetrical physical activity), and track athletes. They found that at the higher speeds (240°/s to 300°/s), differences between preferred and non-preferred leg strength became apparent, and that significant inter-individual differences existed in bilateral mus-

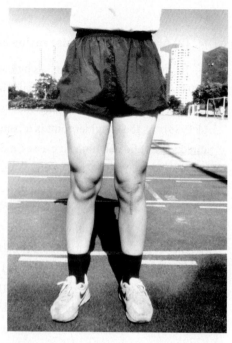

Figure 3-6 Marked decrease in the size of the left thigh in an athlete who underwent an "ACL" operation to the left knee.

cle strength measures. Their data were not corrected for gravity. Read and Bellamy (1990) therefore argued that it should not automatically be assumed that equalizing both sides of the body will prevent injury. The symmetry assumption may be valid in the measurement of all major muscle groups in the lower extremities, but not for many muscle groups in the upper extremities (Kannus 1994). This can be explained by the great effect exerted by dominance in the upper limb. For example, playing tennis will develop the strength of the dominant arm more, while the legs will be stressed more or less equally. The relationship between bilateral muscle imbalance and the occurrence of injury is still controversial and unclear. Figure 3-6 shows an athlete with a distinct discrepancy in limb size, following surgery on the knee.

d. Eccentric/concentric ratio

The production of smooth muscle motion requires concentric contraction of the agonist muscle group to accelerate the limb, while the antagonists generate eccentric work to decelerate the limb, and to control and prevent supraphysiological joint loading. In throwing, the shoulder internal rotators contract eccentrically to decelerate the limb during the cocking phase, while the hamstrings act eccentrically to achieve deceleration of knee extension during sprinting (Perrin 1993). Figure 3-7 illustrates the throwing action with extreme external rotation. Eccentric muscle function also allows lowering of both objects and body weight, besides providing

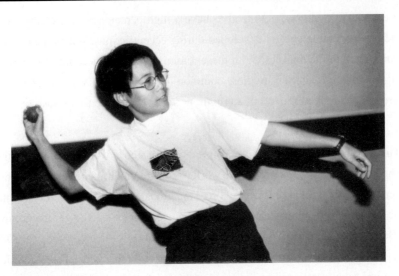

Figure 3-7 Extreme external rotation during a pitching action.

stability (Kramer et al 1993). The concentric maximum moments of the hip, knee and ankle are less than the eccentric moments. Their reciprocal relationship depends on the speed of motion at which a given muscle action is tested (Kellis and Baltzopoulos 1995).

Jonhagen et al (1994) studied hamstring injuries in sprinters, and endorsed the role of concentric and eccentric strength in the development of injuries. It has been suggested that there is no relationship between isokinetic concentric strength of individual muscles and injuries in soccer players (Paton et al 1989), but it has also been suggested that poor eccentric muscle strength of the hamstring group may cause hamstring strains (Stanton and Purdam 1989). Worrell et al (1991) did not find any differences in either concentric or eccentric lower limb muscle torque between injured and uninjured athletes. Their study may have been influenced by the wide variability in sporting background and standard of the subjects. Furthermore, the severity of the injuries reported was moderate, resulting in an average of 2-week absence from training and competition. Posch et al (1989) have suggested that eccentric strength is probably not significantly related to injuries. Jonhagen et al (1994) demonstrated that sprinters who had suffered hamstring tears, requiring average 2-month absence from their sport, were significantly weaker than uninjured sprinters in eccentric contraction of the hamstrings at the three velocities measured (30°/s, 180°/s and 230°/s). The injured athletes also showed weaker concentric contraction at slow speeds. The authors speculated that the contributing factor to the hamstring injuries may have been the poor eccentric hamstring strength, especially during the high angular velocities, common in sprinting.

Lieber and Fridén (1988) have established that after intensive eccentric training, there is predominant disruption of fast fibers. The hamstring group has a high percentage of fast fibers

(Garrett et al 1983), and sprinters tend to have a high percentage of fast fibers (Costill et al 1976). The considerable tension developed during eccentric muscle action can cause high intrinsic forces within the muscles. With these reasons taken into account, it is perhaps not surprising that hamstring injuries are more common in sprinters (Jonhagen et al 1994). Sprinters may therefore need greater levels of strength, not only to be able to run fast, but also to avoid injury.

In daily activities, the agonist muscles produce concentric work to accelerate the limb forward. The antagonists generate eccentric work to control the limb movement and/or to prevent joint overloading. Some authors have reported that imbalance in the ratio of concentric agonist/ eccentric antagonist action may cause inappropriate loading of a given muscle group, leading to injury (Bennet and Stauber 1986). This has not been shown by others (Posch et al 1989, Trudell-Jackson et al 1989). However, limited data are available on this issue. The eccentric reciprocal muscle group ratio is affected by a large number of factors, including age, gender, training status and gravity correction (Kellis and Baltzopoulos 1995). Fast speeds appear to have little effect on eccentric H:Q ratio, in contrast to concentric H:Q ratio, which increases from slow to high speeds (Kellis and Baltzopoulos 1995). Kellis and Baltzopoulos (1995) have indicated that in future it may be more informative to study the eccentric antagonist/concentric agonist ratio as these types of actions occur during daily and athletic activities.

e. Deficits in muscle strength and endurance

The single most commonly used criterion to differentiate between normal and abnormal muscle strength involves contralateral comparison, provided the injury or condition is not bilateral (Sapega 1990). In non-athletes and athletes who do not participate in asymmetrical activities, symmetry is considered the norm for muscles of the lower extremity, but not for the upper extremity (Sapega 1990). Reference values for bilateral and reciprocal strength ratios have been discussed. In general, inter-extremity imbalance in strength in an individual muscle group is taken as a difference of 10% or more (Nunn and Mayhew 1988).

Muscle endurance is defined as the ability of the contracting muscles to perform repeated contractions against a load (Baltzopoulos and Brodie 1989), or as the rate at which a person fatigues during muscular work (Cybex 340 System User's Manual. Lumex Inc., Ronkonkoma. NY11779, USA, 1988). A more detailed definition is given in Section 3. Typically, muscle endurance is expressed in terms of the number of repetitions of a maximum effort test movements that are necessary to reach a 50% reduction in torque output, or as the percent declines in work, torque or power from the beginning to the end of a certain time period, or after a set number of repetitions (Kannus 1994). Twenty-five repetitions are normally sufficient for most joint movements. The Cybex manual recommends a power-endurance test at 180°/s or 240°/s, where endurance is determined by a 50% decrement, from peak power, in a given muscle group (Figures 3-8, 3-9).

Muscle endurance may be tested concentrically or eccentrically, and it is reported that with the eccentric mode of exercise, the decline in peak moment tends to be less, when the angular velocity is fast, from 180°/s to 240°/s (Verdonck et al 1994, Gray and Chandler 1989), than at lower velocities (Kawakami et al 1993, Komi and Viitasalo 1977). For the evaluation of ipsilateral and bilateral muscle strength and endurance, few standard reference values applicable to different groups of people are available. As a rule, data must be specific for the population and the test mode or technique employed (Sapega 1990). Profiling of musculoskeletal performance, especially in athletes, must involve measures of strength, power, endurance, flexibility, and other factors pertinent to performance in the sport of the athlete being investigated (Sapega

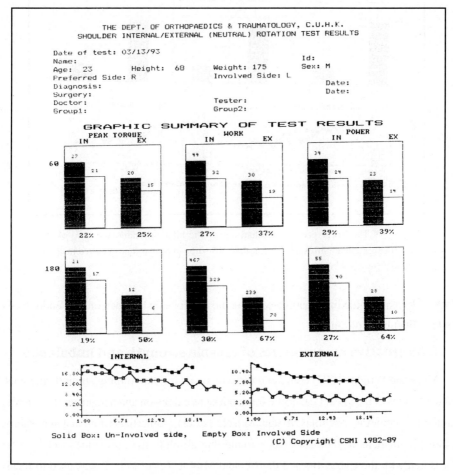

Figure 3-8 A summary chart showing bilateral discrepancies greater than 10% between the involved and the uninvolved limb in terms of peak torque, work and power.

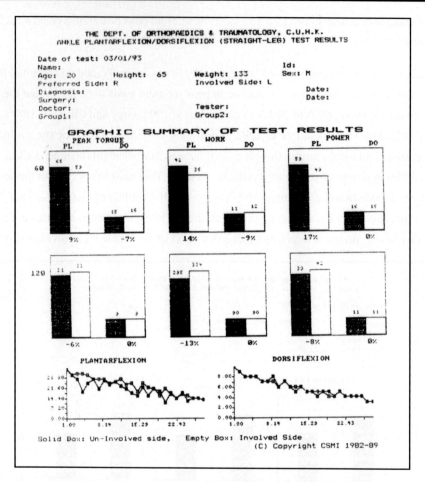

Figure 3-9 The lower part of the chart shows the bilateral endurance ratio of ankle plantarflexors and dorsiflexors. Greater than 50% drop in peak torque occurred in all muscle groups tested.

1990). Currently, little information exists on the relationship between muscle endurance indices and the likelihood of injury.

f. Alternative assessments of muscle strength and imbalance

Moss and Wright (1993) compared three methods for determining strength and muscle imbalance ratios of the knee. Peak force for quadriceps extension and hamstring flexion was measured using isometric (Nicholas Manual Muscle Tester), isoinertial (Universal and Nautilus) and isokinetic methods (Cybex II+). They found that absolute strength values were greater when measured with the Cybex II+ and the Manual Muscle Tester (which was used to measure the eccentric component). The differences were attributed to the specific aspect measured by each mode of testing. Therefore, this data should not be generalized. Similar values for the three different modes of exercise were reported for bilateral strength imbalance ratios for knee extension. The Nautilus produced a lower knee flexion reading. These data were in agreement with Nunn and Mayhew (1988). For ipsilateral strength ratios, similar results were achieved with isometric and isoinertial methods, whereas the isokinetic test produced significantly greater flexion/extension ratios. Again, this was in agreement with the findings of Nunn and Mayhew (1988). Moss and Wright (1993) concluded that absolute strength values were not interchangeable between testing modes, but that, except for the Cybex II+ (ipsilateral) and Nautilus (bilateral knee flexion), strength imbalance ratios could be interchanged.

2. Isokinetics as a diagnostic aid

An isokinetic curve can be used to assist in the diagnosis of injuries and joint pathologies (Figure 3-10). This complements but does not replace formal clinical diagnosis and appropriate investigations. Specific changes in the isokinetic torque curve may be related to certain pathological conditions, such as anterior knee pain (AKP), patella subluxation, musculo-tendinous strains, tendonitis, capsular/ligamentous insufficiency and shoulder impingement. When interpreting isokinetic curves, it is important to bear in mind that a number of confounding factors, such as patient motivation and willingness to comply may influence results. Currently, most available information regarding torque curve interpretation is related to the knee joint. (Please refer to Section 3 for further details on the assessment of torque curves.)

Although the shape of the isokinetic torque curve may be abnormal in various conditions and injuries, the scientific data to support the specificity of this finding are lacking (Sapega 1990). Reproducible and temporary deteriorations in force output during isokinetic assessment

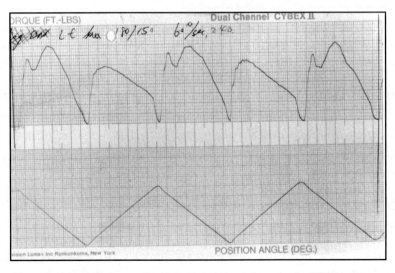

Figure 3-10 Marked abnormality in the knee curve as shown by the CDRC indicates a possible knee pathology.

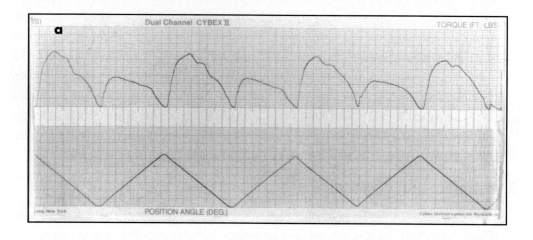

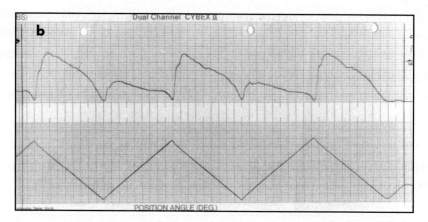

Figure 3-11 These two CDRC graphs illustrate a difference in the range of motion between the two knees tested with the same speed using the same dynamometer. a) a knee with a smaller range of motion; b) a knee with a greater range of motion.

are commonly associated with inhibition by pain over specific portions of the ROM (Davies 1984). However, pain itself should not be regarded as diagnostic or as specific enough to distinguish one type of pathology from another (Sapega 1990). It is also possible that the reduction in ROM may be caused by joint stiffness, or general weakness, originating from muscle atrophy or neural factors (Figure 3-11).

3. Rehabilitation from injury
a. Early rehabilitation

The effects of immobilization were elegantly illustrated in the study by MacDougall et al (1980) where the elbow joint was immobilized for 5 to 6 weeks. The experiment involved either training followed by 5 to 6 weeks of immobilization or vice versa. Under both sets of conditions, the slow fiber area (type I) decreased by 27% and the fast fiber area (type II) by 35%. A concomitant 41% decrement in measured isokinetic strength was noted. Pre-training did not alter the muscle's susceptibility to atrophy and decreased performance. Other factors that may influence the type and degree of muscle atrophy include joint capsule edema (whether injury or surgery-related), and damage to the innervation of the capsule (Sherman et al 1982). Gydikov (1976) and Eriksson (1981) have shown that even mild pain may inhibit the monosynaptic reflexes to type I fibers and related motor units, while severe pain inhibits these reflexes to both type I and type II fibers and their corresponding motor units.

Early mobilization is therefore indicated following injury or surgery (DeCarlo et al 1992, Shelbourne and Nitz 1990, Sherman et al 1982, Salter et al 1980, Eriksson and Haggmark 1979, Costill et al 1977). After major knee ligamentous surgery the advantages of an early mobiliza-tion program include curtailing the effects of disuse, avoiding capsular contractures, maintain-ing articular cartilage nutrition, and allowing early controlled forces on growing collagen tis-sues (Noyes et al 1987). A delicate balance must be achieved in the early phases of rehabilita-tion. On the one hand, mobilization may increase articular edema and swelling, and may pro-mote joint effusion (Noyes et al 1987), as well as damage the healing tissues. On the other hand, traditional post-operative programs involving overprotection and immobilization may seriously increase the risk of cartilage damage, joint contracture, stiffness and associated tightness of peripatellar tissues (Shelbourne and Nitz 1990, Noyes et al 1987).

Isokinetic exercises have been used extensively in the rehabilitation of injuries, and a large body of literature now exists evaluating its efficacy, especially in the rehabilitation of the knee. As pain, joint stiffness, contractures and muscle weakness often limit the joint ROM, exercises must be safe and avoid undue stress on the given joint. In this respect, isokinetic exercises have advantages and disadvantages. One of the main advantages is the variable resistance equal to the applied force that isokinetic devices offer. It is possible to exercise the joint through the full ROM, with safe levels of resistance at points where muscle weakness or pain occurs, and upper limit to the speed of muscular movement. Also, no return of limb-lever arm is required, avoid-ing potentially damaging eccentric contractions (Perrin 1993). Active isokinetic dynamometers can also provide CPM. This has obvious advantages in early rehabilitation of major injuries, as joint movement is possible without the forces that naturally occur with muscle contractions. O'Driscoll and Salter (1983) studied the effects of CPM on the clearance of hemarthrosis from a synovial joint in the rabbit. They found that the rate of clearance was more than twice as fast with CPM than with cast immobilization. Significantly less blood remained in the synovium after one week with CPM and less trapping of erythrocytes was also noted. From a patient's view point, isokinetic devices offer valuable feedback on his/her progress, both visually (by looking at the shape of the torque curve) and quantitatively (torque values attained for PT and endurance) (Figure 3-12). This can be of particular help providing motivation for the athlete whose rehabilitation is often a long-term process. Isokinetic exercises may have limited benefits in the early rehabilitation of joints with a restricted ROM such as the ankle joint after Achilles tendon repair. Osternig (1986) points out that as isokinetic dynamometers require an acceleration phase before resistance is applied to the exercising muscle group, it is possible that the period of stress is insufficient, and hence the exercise ineffective when the arc of motion is limited. In such cases, the limb must be accelerated fast to produce resistance throughout the desired range, otherwise loading will occur only during the latter parts of the range of motion (Davis 1984). Also, when training a muscle group through a small arc of movement, slow velocities must be applied in order to allow the contractile components of the muscles to develop

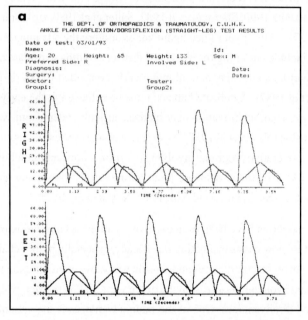

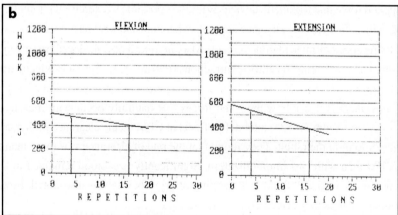

Figure 3-12 a) A graphic report showing strength as peak torque, and the ranges of motion of the tested joints. b) A graphic report showing the work endurance ratios of the normal knee muscles tested.

their fullest capacity (Osternig 1986), and speeds ranging from 60°/s to 180°/s have been recommended (Davis 1984). Because of this difficulty with short arc movements, isokinetic exercises may need supplementation with isometric exercises, performed at multiple angles, and at 20° intervals (Osternig 1986). Isometric exercises may also be performed with an isokinetic dynamometer set at zero velocity.

After rehabilitation, atrophy may still be present despite normal measured strength. It is essential to remember that strength gains are not dependent on muscle size, as neural factors play an important part (McDonagh et al 1983, Sherman et al 1982, Ikai and Fukunaga 1970). Although there is a strong correlation between muscle cross-sectional area and its potential for producing force, a more efficient activation of motor units in response to strength training has been demonstrated during maximum effort in EMG studies. Muscle strength depends on the number of motor units activated and their frequency of contraction. During strength training, there is an increase in the number of motor units and number of fibers per motor unit recruited with increasing loads. As the load increases, the principal mechanism for the development of force is increased rate of firing (Astrand and Rodahl 1986). This impulse traffic reaching the motor neurons is important, especially in the less well trained subjects. It appears in most situations that maximal voluntary effort does not engage all the motor units of the active muscle at tetanic frequencies. Inhibition of varying degrees exists in some motor neurons, depending on supraspinal and proprioceptor activity. Such inhibition is reduced (or facilitation is increased) with training, and the muscle mass can be used more effectively in the contraction (Astrand and Rodahl 1986). With isokinetic training, neural and biochemical adaptations appear to be responsible for much of the improvement in strength (Esselman et al 1991, Ewing et al 1990, Cote et al 1988).

b. Functional rehabilitation

While most research work with isokinetic dynamometers has been performed with the knee joint, isokinetic rehabilitation of other joints, such as the ankle and the shoulder, is becoming more common. Testing and exercising of the trunk has also been made possible with the development of appropriate devices (Figure 3-13). The following paragraphs will review the available research literature on the efficacy and problems of isokinetics in rehabilitation. The use of concentric and eccentric modes will also be evaluated.

(1) Mode of exercise in rehabilitation

One of the most comprehensive studies on mode of exercise was conducted by Timm (1988). He collated data on 5,381 patients over a 5-year period to evaluate the effectiveness of four rehabilitation programs after a variety of surgical procedures on the knee, none of them involving the ACL. Although well controlled, this study was retrospective and lacked procedural randomization, which to some extent limited its validity. The four rehabilitation programs

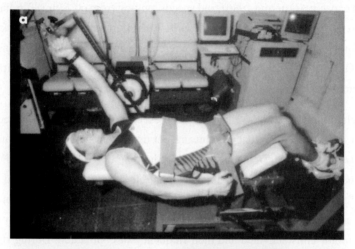

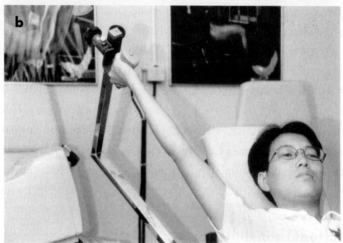

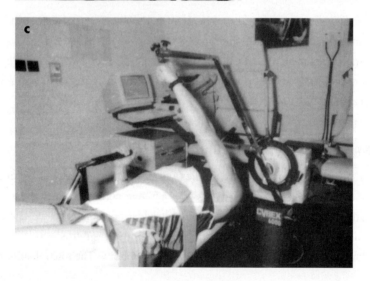

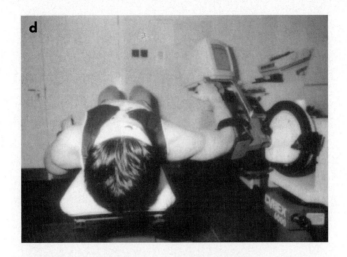

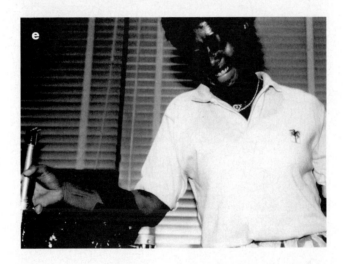

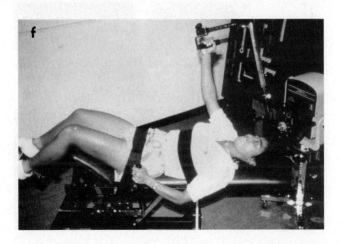

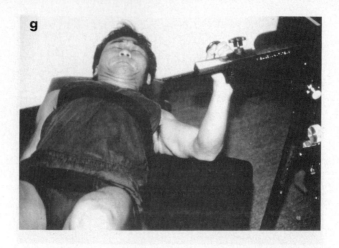

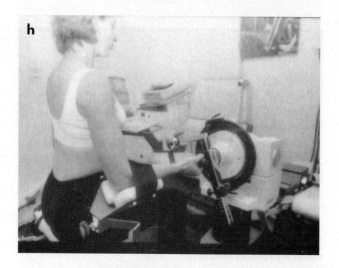

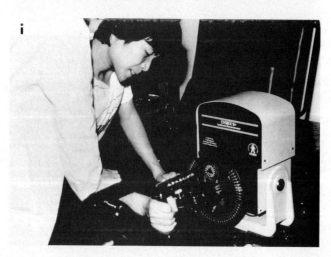

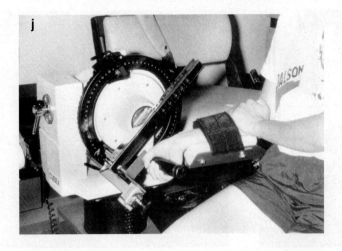

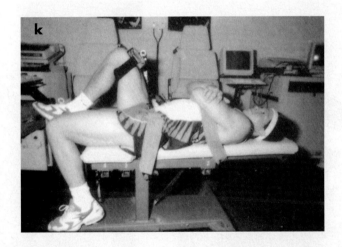

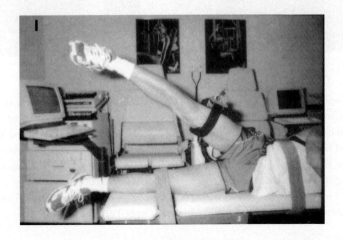

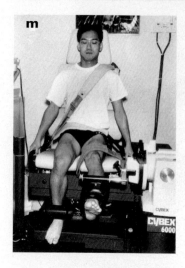
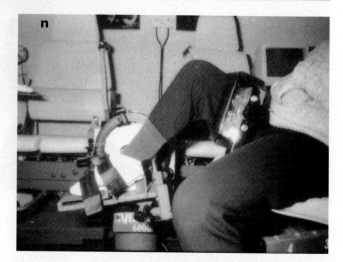
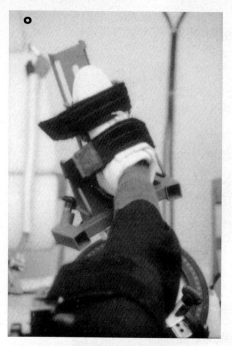
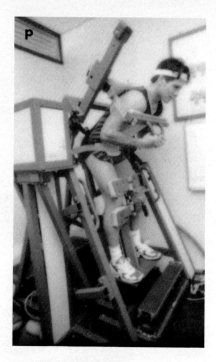

Figure 3-13 Testing of the major joints in various planes. a) testing of shoulder flexion/extension; b) testing of shoulder abduction/adduction; c) testing of shoulder horizontal abduction/adduction; d) testing of shoulder internal/external rotation with shoulder at 90° abduction; e) testing of shoulder internal/external rotation in neutral position; f) testing of shoulder PNF pattern. Note that the UBXT is at an angle with the dynamometer to obtain the desired effect; g) testing of elbow flexion/extension; h) testing of forearm supination/pronation; i) testing of wrist radial/ulnar deviation; j) testing of wrist flexion/extension; k) testing of hip flexion/extension; l) testing of hip abduction/adduction; m) testing of knee flexion/extension; n) testing of ankle dorsiflexion/plantarflexion; o) testing of ankle inversion/eversion; p) testing of trunk flexion/extension using the Cybex TEF unit.

were: 1) no exercise, 2) home exercises (instructions on isometrics and calisthenics but without supervision), 3) isoinertial exercises (incorporating isometrics and calisthenics with supervision) and 4) isokinetic exercises (incorporating all aforementioned cycle ergometry and proprioceptive exercises, advancing to isokinetic training). The criterion for success was resumption of required activities without recurrence of symptoms. The results suggested that the isokinetic program was more effective and efficient than the other methods. Discharge was quicker: 8.9 weeks instead of an average of 10 weeks for the home program, and 12.3 weeks for the isoinertial program. Although the study is extremely informative, it is difficult to distinguish between the specific effects of the different types of exercises adopted. Also, the cumulative effect of the various types of training may have influenced the outcome. Grimby et al (1980) also investigated the effectiveness of structured isokinetic training, weight training and self-training following ACL surgery. Those who underwent isokinetic training showed a complete restoration of bilateral strength symmetry at all velocities. They also showed greater strength gains. Isokinetic training has also been evaluated for the treatment of patella tendinitis (Jensen and Fabio 1989), medial collateral and anterior and posterior cruciate ligament injury (Burnie and Brodie 1986) and post-meniscectomy (Jensen and Fabio 1989). Sherman et al (1982) evaluated a regime of isokinetic and isoinertial rehabilitation, and found that the isokinetic mode was superior. These studies have demonstrated the merits of isokinetics over other modes of exercise in the rehabilitation of the knee joint. However, negative aspects of isokinetic training in knee joint rehabilitation have recently emerged. Knee extension produces large compression forces on the involved joints during maximal contractions. This may put undue stress on the ligaments (Kaufman et al 1991, Nisell et al 1989), leading to delayed tissue healing, especially in cartilage defect as pain limitation of the movement in these cases is not always effective (Kannus 1994). Different modes of muscle training in the rehabilitation of other joints than the knee are currently lacking.

Isokinetic machines have become increasingly popular in the rehabilitation setting. Commonly, clinicians and therapists involved in isokinetic rehabilitation believe them to be superior to traditional resistance training methods. Surprisingly, no prospective study has compared the effects of isoinertial and isokinetic conditioning in the rehabilitation of soft musculoskeletal tissues injuries (Morrisey et al 1995). Studies suggest that isokinetic exercise may be superior for functional performance, although the evidence is controversial.

(2) Specificity of training speed

In functional rehabilitation, and especially in the rehabilitation of athletes, it is important to consider specificity of velocity in conditioning. The old concept of speed specificity has been challenged, although it is generally accepted that the velocity of training should be close to the actual velocities required in daily living and in sporting actions. All fiber types may be recruited in a maximum effort in a slow contraction against a high resistance, as well as in a fast contraction, at lower resistance (Astrand and Rodahl 1986). The velocity specific effects of training on muscle strength have been reported for normal subjects (Coyle et al 1981). It is of practical interest in rehabilitation and in sports, whether the effects of training at a given velocity will be transferable to other velocities. Most studies have found a velocity "overflow" effect. Muscle performance is improved not only at the training velocity, but at velocities above and below it. Timm (1987) found an overflow effect to both slower and faster speeds with isokinetic training at 120°/s. Davies et al (1986) and Timm (1987) reported a bi-directional overflow of $\pm 60°/s$ from a velocity of 180°/s for quadriceps performance, but not for the hamstrings. Parker (1982) has proposed that the appropriate rehabilitation velocity can be determined according to the condition of the injured limb determined by isometric assessment. Sherman et al (1982) recommended velocities ranging from 60°/s to 300°/s, whereas Grimby (1985) stated that the velocity should be guided by the phase of rehabilitation, type and degree of muscular hypotrophy and individual reaction. More recently it has been suggested that a velocity differential of 90°/s may be used in isokinetic conditioning programs (Dvir 1995).

(3) Open versus closed kinetic chain conditioning

Open kinetic chain (OKC) (Figure 3-14a) refers to distal-end-free positions involving non-weight-bearing positions, such as knee extension. OKC exists when the peripheral joint of the extremity can move freely, such as waving a hand (Palmitier et al 1991).

Closed kinetic chain (CKC) (Figure 3-14b) refers to distal-end-fixed positions, involving weight-bearing positions, such as the squat. A CKC thus exists when the foot meets resistance. For example the swing phase of gait involves the foot in an OKC state but as soon as the foot strikes the ground, a CKC is formed (Palmitier et al 1991).

The terms OKC and CKC describe temporary set-up of the joints or body segments. The two positions are illustrated in Figure 3-14. Interest in OKC and CKC exercises in rehabilitation relates to the establishment of optimum training protocols. Closed kinetic chain exercises are weight-bearing and lead to joint compression, which theoretically adds stability to the joint (Bynum et al 1995). The stresses placed on the limb also act to prevent muscle and bone atrophy and to improve proprioception (Bynum et al 1995). In OKC exercises, the foot is free, and thus less compression and larger shear forces are exerted across the joint (Bynum et al 1995). It is important for the clinician and the therapist to determine a right balance between the two kinds of exercises in order to accelerate recovery from injury or surgery.

(a) Rehabilitation with OKC or CKC?

The human body functions in a complex way, incorporating both OKC and CKC actions each closely following the other. From a functional point of view both types of kinetic chain exercises might be included in a rehabilitation program. Henning et al (1985) were the first to

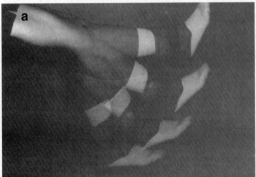

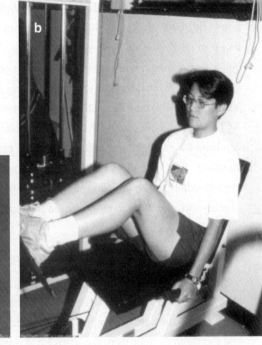

Figure 3-14 a) An open kinetic chain exercise. b) A closed kinetic chain exercise.

suggest that, in vivo, isometric knee extension at $0°$ and $22°$ produced five to seventeen times more strain on the ACL than weight-bearing exercises such as stationary cycling, rope jumping, half squats with one leg or level-ground walking. Solomonow et al (1987) showed that a protective reflex exists between the ACL and hamstrings. When the ACL is overloaded, a reflex contraction of the hamstrings occurs, protecting the ligament. This reflex is recruited during isokinetic knee extension testing. Solomonow et al (1987) concluded that isokinetic testing may be contraindicated in ACL reconstructed knees. Such overloading in normal knees is yet to be examined. Shelbourne and Nitz (1990) studied the effects of CKC exercises as a part of accelerated rehabilitation post ACL reconstruction where weight-bearing started on Day 1 after the operation. They found CKC exercises significantly more effective in returning the patients back to normal function. Accelerated rehabilitation with CKC exercises led to full functioning and sports participation in 4 to 6 months after reconstruction, while it took 9 to 12 months with traditional methods. Shelbourne and Nitz (1990) suggested that CKC exercises place functional stresses on the joint similar to normal weight-bearing activities. Thus, CKC exercises provide stability and perhaps a more strenuous strengthening workout without the degree of shear forces that occur with OKC exercises. Such shear forces are kept lower due to larger compressive forces and the coactivation of the hamstrings group, which act as joint stabilizers (Solomonow et al 1987). In some cases though, CKC exercises may exert higher shear loads than submaximal isokinetic exercises. In the long-term, Shelbourne and Nitz (1990) have found no complications with CKC exercises. Interestingly, they also reported that motivation was an essential factor in rehabilitation success, as highly motivated athletes were able to gain initial levels of quadriceps strength within 10 weeks of the operation. Ohkoshi et al (1991) showed with EMG analysis that the mean shear force in standing subjects was posterior at all knee flexion angles. Yack et al (1993) and Drez et al (1992) reported significantly less anterior tibial translation in ACL-deficient knees with CKC exercises, compared with OKC exercises. Bynum et al (1995) conducted a prospective randomized study on OKC versus CKC exercises after ACL reconstruction. CKC exercises appear to be safe and effective. Accelerated rehabilitation emphasizing immediate full motion and early weight-bearing and strength training reduced the incidence of post-operative flexion or extension loss and patellafemoral pain without any major negative side effects.

(b) CKC exercise and isokinetic training

Most isokinetic exercises are by definition OKC, but because the limb, for example the leg when testing the knee, is strapped to the lever arm and the thigh is stabilized, the exercise is sometimes considered to be CKC (Dvir 1995) (Figure 3-15). However, as such exercises do induce compression on the given joint, we feel that to call them CKC is unwarranted. CKC exercises also train proprioception, which is not the case when limbs are merely strapped into a given position. Cybex, however, has developed an isokinetic stepping machine which operates on the CKC principle and Biodex and Kin-Com, for example, have new CKC attachments. These can be used in all exercise modes (active, passive, eccentric etc) and allow changes in speed, torque and ROM. Little information is currently available on CKC isokinetic exercises.

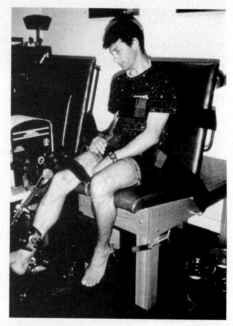

Figure 3-15 Isokinetic knee exercise. A Velcro is strapped round the thigh just above the knee.

(4) Eccentric training in rehabilitation

Eccentric muscle actions are an integral part of athletic and daily activities. Lowering the body, lowering a heavy object and running downhill involve eccentric actions. At any given joint velocity, the maximum possible moment the muscle is able to exert is generated through eccentric acions. The mechanism for this is still somewhat unclear (Kellis and Baltzopoulos 1995), but a cross-bridge detachment mechanism different from that during concentric actions has been postulated. During eccentric contractions no energy is required for detachment, yet the cross-bridges are exerting greater force. The elastic components of the muscle may provide additional force during eccentric actions (Cabri 1991).

Most research has centered on the clinical use of isokinetic concentric exercise, and less is known about the effects of isokinetic eccentric exercise regimes. The mode specificity of both concentric and eccentric training is controversial (Kellis and Baltzopoulos 1995). Dvir (1995) concluded that concentric training results both in enhanced concentric and eccentric strength gains, whereas eccentric training results in eccentric gains only. Thus the former would be non-specific, and the latter specific in their effects. Because different protocols were employed in these studies, it is premature to make definitive conclusions.

Isokinetic eccentric exercise programs have been evaluated by few investigators. Jensen and Fabio (1989) analyzed the effects of quadriceps femoris muscle eccentric training program on strength gains in patients with patellar tendinitis. Although not statistically significant, training leads to an increase in the eccentric quadriceps femoris muscle work capacity over the 8-week period (Jensen and Fabio 1989). They concluded that eccentric exercise may be effective in the treatment of patella tendinitis, but that knee pain may limit strength gains. Stanish et al (1986) studied the effectiveness of eccentric exercise in the rehabilitation of chronic tendonitis. They prescribed a regime of eccentric exercise, stretching, and ice with favorable results, and proposed that strength training should be specific to the task of the tendon. Bennet and Stauber (1986) used eccentric exercise three times a week to treat anterior knee pain caused by vastus medialis weakness, and concluded that the condition was associated with a deficit in eccentric moment. The validity of their findings was later questioned (Trudell-Jackson et al 1989).

Eccentric training may be beneficial to patients with limited exercise capacity because eccentric work is associated with lower metabolic cost and greater strength development compared with concentric work (Dean 1988). Kellis and Baltzopoulos (1995) suggested that eccentric training may also be beneficial in the rehabilitation of muscles which often work eccentrically, for example, the hamstrings.

(5) Acute cardiovascular effects associated with isokinetic exercise

Cardiocirculatory responses to isokinetic exercise have not been widely studied. Such responses have implications for patients with cardiac disease and circulatory problems. It is important to know whether precautions need to be taken prior to commencing an isokinetic training program. (Rantanen et al 1995, Horstmann et al 1994, Scharf et al 1994, Eckhardt et al 1991). Horstmann et al (1994) studied the cardiocirculatory responses to isokinetic exercise in 64 males aged between 22 and 60. They found that increase in heart rate was most pronounced after concentric exercise, followed by eccentric and isometric exercise. No age-relationship was found in heart rate responses. The most pronounced increase in systolic blood pressure was recorded after concentric exercise, followed by eccentric, and then isometric exercise. Again, no age-dependence was found. Conversely, diastolic blood pressure demonstrated a slight fall in all forms of exercise. Horstmann et al (1994) concluded that no special precautions are required prior to isokinetic exercise. Scharf et al (1994) compared metabolic and hemodynamic changes in 21 healthy young men during isokinetic and ergometric loading. They found that heart rate and blood pressure were higher during isokinetic loading, and concluded that isokinetic testing may be dangerous for patients with cardiocirculatory disturbances. The heart rate and blood pressure values reported for isokinetic exercise in this study, though significantly different from those derived during ergometry, were not unduly alarming. Ekhardt et al (1991) also reported markedly elevated blood pressure and heart rate responses to isokinetic exercise and advocated caution with isokinetic testing. Heart rate responses to isokinetic trunk strength testing were also investigated by Rantanen et al (1995). They found that cardiovascular capacity was an important factor, limiting performance in isokinetic testing of patients with neck and low back pain, especially at higher speeds. Rantanen et al (1995) concluded that patients with suspected cardiac problems need special attention.

Acute cardiovascular stress during weight training can be high. During the performance of a two-legged leg press to failure at 95% of one repetition maximum, in which a Valsalva maneuver was allowed, pressures of 320/250mmHg and a heart rate of 170 beats per minute have been reported (MacDougall et al 1985). Sale et al (1993) compared the blood pressure responses to a single maximal leg press action on an isokinetic device and a weight training machine. They found that peak systolic and diastolic pressures observed during weightlifting were significantly higher than during isokinetic exercise. They concluded that resisted leg press actions cause extreme elevations in blood pressure. The degree of voluntary effort rather than the type of muscle action employed was the major determinant of blood pressure response. In summary, 3 of 4 investigators advocated precautionary measures prior to embarking on isokinetic testing and training programs. Such precautions are standard with traditional weight training, especially for non-athletes.

B. Isokinetics in Sports Science

The development of any training program needs to take into account the basic principles of training, including specificity, overload and reversibility (Astrand and Rodahl 1986). To produce a noticeable training effect, exercise stress has to be of sufficient intensity, duration and frequency, and for optimum gains, stress should be increased periodically. Just as important for the sports performer is the specificity of the training stimulus (Astrand and Rodahl 1986). The aim of strength training in sports is to gain improvements in functional performance. Aspects of specificity which require particular consideration involve the mode and the speed of exercise.

The mode of exercise specificity involves consideration of the role of static and dynamic strength in the given sport, such as the hand grip in windsurfing (static), jumping in steeplechase (dynamic), or a mix of both, needed by a gymnast. It is common for coaches to prescribe resistance training which reproduces the actual movement patterns required in the sporting action, such as the hand stroke in freestyle. This enhances the development of optimal neuromuscular adaptations. Evaluation of the movement patterns involved will indicate whether concentric or eccentric actions should be emphasized. The speed at which the movement occurs in the actual sport is typically simulated during training. Finally, the need for assessment of strength and power in sport is fourfold:

Assessment of strength and power are carried out to:
1) Quantify the relative significance of strength and power in specific sports;
2) Detect areas of weakness which may subsequently be improved;
3) Identify talent; and
4) Monitor the effects of training.

Muscle function tests should be closely related to performance. They should discriminate effectively between individuals of differing performance levels, and be capable of detecting training induced changes in performance. Studies evaluating currently used tests of muscle function disagree on their capacity to satisfy the requirements outlined above. There are data to suggest that both isokinetic (Alexander 1989, Perrine and Edgerton 1975) and isometric (Häkkinen et al 1986, Viitasalo and Aura 1984) tests are strongly related to performance, and conversely that the relationship does not exist (Young and Bilby 1993, Komi et al 1982). Abe et al (1992), Oberg et al (1986), Mero et al (1981), Gillam et al (1979) found that isometric and isokinetic tests can be used to discriminate between individuals of differing performance levels, while a number of authors reported the contrary about isokinetic (Fry et al 1991, Hurley et al 1988) and isometric tests (Abe et al 1992, Fry et al 1991). Few studies have assessed the ability of the different tests to monitor training induced changes in performance (Wilson and Murphy 1995). Among clinicians who treat musculoskeletal injuries, there is a strong belief that isokinetic exercises may be superior to traditional weight training in improving muscle strength (Timm 1988). In the following paragraphs, the efficacy of isokinetic dynamometry, related to testing and training of athletes and uninjured subjects, will be examined.

1. Isokinetics as a training tool
a. Isokinetics versus weight training

The results from the study by Pipes and Wilmore (1975) have been widely quoted to support the superiority of isokinetics as a training tool. The validity of this study has since been seriously questioned (Wilmore 1979). Four other investigations have been carried out since, with mixed results. Pearson and Costill (1988), Meadors et al (1983), Davies (1977) found that weight training was significantly more effective than isokinetic exercise in improving weight-lifting performance. Gettman et al (1980) found no differences in the training effects of the two modes of exercise. The specificity of training effects and the importance of assessing them using the same exercise mode as in training is highlighted in the studies, which compared isokinetic strength changes resulting from weight training and isokinetic training. Of six studies (Pearson and Costill 1988, Smith and Melton 1981, Gettman et al 1980, Davies 1977, Moffroid et al 1969, Thistle et al 1967), only Davies (1977) found that weight training was more effective in improving isokinetic performance. Gettman et al (1980) found that isokinetic training improved isokinetic leg press performance by 42%, whereas weight training only improved isokinetic performance by 17%.

b. Isokinetics and functional performance

As already mentioned, in the sporting context it is vital that the time and effort invested in resistance training be translated into functional improvement. Smith and Melton (1981) trained the knee extensors and flexors of three groups of athletes: one group with weights (n=3), another group isokinetically at slow velocities (30°/s, 60°/s and 90°/s) (n=3), and a third one isokinetically at fast velocities (180°/s to 300°/s) (n=3). They evaluated changes in vertical jump height, broad jump distance, and a 40-yard dash time. Vertical jump increases in the three groups were 2%, 4%, and 5% respectively. The fast isokinetic group showed a 9% improvement in the broad jump, a 10% improvement in the 40-yard dash, whereas the weight training and slow velocity isokinetic groups improved only by 1%. This study suggests that fast isokinetic training may be superior to weight training in improving motor performance. It does not, however, offer conclusive evidence. Sample sizes were small, there were no formal statistical analyses, and there were slight but important differences in the exercise protocols adopted in the weight training and isokinetic groups.

c. Speed specificity and isokinetics

Speed specificity during concentric isokinetic training has been investigated in various studies (see Morrissey et al 1995 for a review). However, only two have assessed this aspect with weight training (Young and Bilby 1993, Palmieri 1987). The specificity of speed of isokinetic training has been studied in relation to both concentric and eccentric muscle activity, and to functional performance. PT is often used as the criterion when assessing the specificity of speed although some feel that angle-specific torque (AST) may be a better indicator of strength gain after a program of isokinetic training as it accounts for the length of the muscle at the point when PT occurs. The use of PT, average force, AST and power as criteria in the assessment of the effectiveness of an isokinetic program will be discussed in relation to speed specificity in isokinetic training.

PT as criterion

One of the fundamental studies on speed specificity was conducted by Moffroid and Whipple (1990). They trained the knee extensors of two groups (n=10 +10) at either 36°/s or 108°/s, and then tested isokinetic strength at 18°/s, 36°/s, 54°/s, 72°/s, 90°/s and 108°/s. They demonstrated that both groups improved performance at and below the training velocity, with the "fast" group improving by 10% or more at all other test velocities as well. These findings were subsequently supported by Costill et al (1979) and Lesmes et al (1978), who found significant strength improvements at and below the 180°/s training velocity, but not at higher test velocities (240°/s and 300°/s). Coyle et al (1981) found some evidence to suggest that strength gains may be made at velocities higher than the training velocity: training at 60°/s resulted in improved performance at 180°/s. They also reported that training at 300°/s significantly increased strength, by at least 15%, at all test speeds employed (0°/s, 60°/s, 180°/s and 300°/s). A number of studies have found incomplete or no carryover of PT gains to velocities below the concentric isokinetic training velocity (Perrin et al 1989, Petersen et al 1989, Smith and Melton 1981). Still, another group of studies have reported little consistency in the degree of training effect on speeds, other than the training velocities employed (Behm and Sale 1993, Bell et al 1989, Garnica 1986) (Figure 3-16).

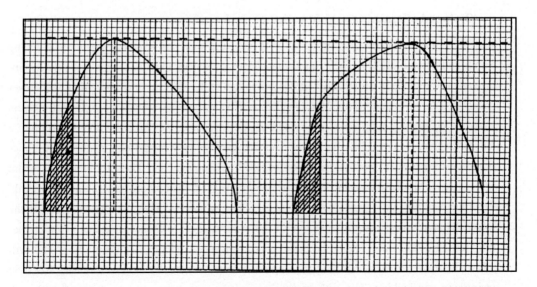

Figure 3-16 Peak torque (PT) at two different angles. The diagram on the left shows PT at an earlier point.

Average force, AST and power as criteria

When average force was used as the outcome measure, Duncan et al (1989) found little or no specificity, as significant strength increases were induced at all three testing velocities in response to eccentric training at 120°/s. Angle-specific torque may be a more appropriate strength criterion than PT, because it partially corrects the possible discrepancies between test speeds. It also equalizes the effects that the length of the muscle and its lever arm will have subsequent results. Particularly in fast isokinetic testing, PT is not reached early in the movement because several degrees of rotation are required to reach the programmed speed (Morrissey et al 1995). Caiozzo et al (1981) reported that strength increases occur both above and below training speeds when measured in terms of AST. They also indicated that higher training speeds were more specific than slower ones. Kanehisa and Miyashita (1983) found that when power was used as the strength criterion, the experimental group, which were trained at 60°/s and 180°/s, showed wider increases in average power than a group trained at 300°/s, which had significant increases only when tested at 240°/s and 300°/s. Both Garnica (1986) and Ewing et al (1990) found that average power changes occurred at slower speeds but not at faster speeds.

(1) Isokinetic eccentric training and speed specificity

Eccentric isokinetic training may not be velocity-specific. Ryan et al (1991) trained the knee flexors of 34 women at 120°/s. Both concentric and eccentric strength increased, when tested at 60°/s, 120°/s and 180°/s. The only exception was concentric action at 60°/s. Mean percent change ranged from 17% to 26%, and the greatest changes were seen at the higher training speeds.

(2) Speed of training and functional performance

The relationship between training velocity and functional performance was investigated by Smith and Melton (1981). They found that the faster speeds (180°/s, 240°/s and 300°/s) improved performance in broad and vertical jumps and in the 40-yard dash more than the slower speeds (30°/s, 60°/s and 90°/s). Van Oteghen (1973) trained two groups of volleyball players with the leg press. Both groups improved their performance over that of a control group to a similar degree. It is possible that faster exercise speed is more beneficial in improving functional performance in sports which require fast body movements. The data however remain inconclusive. Mookerjee et al (1995) investigated the relationship between isokinetic strength, flexibility and the flutter kick speed in female college swimmers. They concluded that PT in the lower extremity plays a significant role in flutter kicking performance, and that velocity-specific testing of the knees should be done in excess of 6.00 rad/s (3.14 rads = 180°). This will allow the dynamometer to mimic the angular velocities actually achieved during freestyle swimming and kicking. The authors emphasized the importance of speed-specific strength training, again in excess of 6.00 rads/s.

(3) Speed specificity and weight training

Young and Bilby (1993) and Palmieri (1987) assessed the effect of two different speeds of training on maximal squat lift and maximum vertical jump. Both studies concluded that weight training, independent of speed, produced significant improvements in the variables measured.

d. Neural and morphological effects of isokinetic training

The maximal force developed by a muscle is related to its cross-sectional area (Astrand and Rodahl 1986). However, during the first few weeks of strength training, particularly in untrained subjects, measurable improvements can be seen in the absence of muscle hypertrophy. This is mainly due to neural adaptations (Enoka 1988). Increased neural activation during strength training is associated with improved synchronization of motor units, an increase in the number of active motor units, and/or their rate of firing (Sale 1992).

A number of studies of morphological changes associated with concentric isokinetic strength training have been published. Cote et al (1988) trained 23 sedentary subjects over a 10-week period using concentric quadriceps contractions. A 54% strength increase was recorded in the absence of changes to the muscle cross-sectional area. Muscle biopsies showed significant increase in percent of type II fiber number and area, although overall fiber area did not increase. These findings were contradicted to Ewing et al (1990), who found no muscle hypertrophy in response to concentric isokinetic strength training, but reported significant increases in the area of type I and II fibers. Coyle et al (1981) reported an increase in the area of type II fibers following fast velocity (300°/s) training, while no increase in type II fiber area was found in the slow (60°/s) training group. Esselman et al (1991) found no significant changes to fiber area after a 12-week isokinetic training program using untrained healthy men. Like Cote et al (1988), Esselman et al (1991) found significant increases in muscle glycolytic (PFK) and mitochondrial (SDH and MDH) enzyme activity. There were also differences in the time pattern of torque gains. Training at 360°/s, which allows greater torque development than fast isokinetic training, showed consistent, steady gains throughout an 8-week period, whereas the fast group (108°/s) reached a plateau after 4 weeks of the 12-week training period. Esselman et al (1991) suggested that the pattern observed was consistent with neural factors resulting in torque gains early in training. The lack of improvement during the remainder of the 12-week program, coupled with the absemce of muscle hypertrophy, indicated that muscle adaptation was not responsible for most of the torque gains measured. Esselman et al (1991) also showed considerable contralateral strength gains. They concluded that neural factors, including improved recruitment and increased synchrony, among others, may have been responsible. They also highlighted that, for sports training, slow speed isokinetic exercise would probably contribute to optimal performance. Their study was unique in that a strong incentive system (payment per torque) was used to ensure that maximum torque was produced in training and testing. In summary, conflicting results have been reported regarding speed specificity in improving sporting performance. Fast isokinetic training was found to be more effective by Van Oteghen et al (1973) and Smith and Melton (1983), whereas Esselman et al (1991) found that slow speed training was more effective. The former involved lower limb training; the latter involved upper limb. Isokinetic strength training does not appear to lead to muscle hypertrophy. Rather, neural and biochemical adaptations seem to contribute to the improvements observed.

Differences in sample size, muscle fiber type distribution, training protocols adopted (Baltzopoulos and Brodie 1989), methods used to determine histological changes (Dvir 1995), and the training status of the subjects may all have influenced the results obtained.

e. Effects of eccentric isokinetic training

There are conflicting findings regarding the effectiveness of eccentric training. Mont et al (1994) and Ellenbecker et al (1988) investigated the effects of eccentric training on functional performance in tennis. Ellenbecker et al (1988) found that eccentric training (velocity spectrum pyramidal ordering: 60°/s, 180°/s, 210°/s, 210°/s, 180°/s, and 60°/s) twice a week, for 6 weeks, did not result in statistically significant strength gains. Neither did eccentric training translate into improved functional performance in terms of the tennis serve: in fact half of the subjects showed a drop in speed of service. Conversely, a systematic increase was seen with concentric training. Mont et al (1994) found an 11% increase in both eccentric and concentric strength, paralleled by an equal increase in average serve velocity. Indeed the serve speed of the eccentric group improved slightly more than that of the concentric group. They found that the training regime (three times per week velocity spectrum pyramidal order training for 6 weeks) promoted service endurance and reduced service variability, which can be important in a prolonged tennis match. Tomberlin et al (1991) reported that isokinetic eccentric training at 100°/s for 6 weeks resulted in significant improvements of eccentric PT and total work, but not in concentric variables. Higbie et al (1994) found that a 10-week eccentric training program improved concentric and eccentric isokinetic strength of the knee extensor muscles by 6.8% and 36.2%, respectively. Concentric training was related to 18.4% and 12.8% improvements in concentric and eccentric performance, respectively.

Eccentric exercise is associated with some negative effects, mainly muscle soreness. Amongst others, Fridén et al (1983) found that an 8-week eccentric cycling program resulted in slight improvements in concentric strength of the knee extensors, but eccentric work capacity improved by 375%. Muscle soreness, associated strength reduction and myofibrillar damage were reduced after prolonged eccentric training. Muscles soreness and damage lead to decreased strength levels, which seem to recover more rapidly after the initial bout of eccentric exercise (Golden and Dudley 1992). Adaptation may already occur before full recovery and restoration of muscle function following an initial eccentric exercise bout (Fridén et al 1983).

Strength improvements associated with eccentric exercise have been attributed to changes in the contractile elements of muscle tissue, and to preferential recruitment of type II, particularly type IIb, fibers, indicating improved coordination. Improved storage of elastic energy and reorganization of the contractile apparatus of muscle fibers together with enzymatic adaptations have been seen with eccentric training (Fridén et al 1983). Changes in connective tissue have also been implicated (Duncan et al 1989). Tomberlin et al (1991) suggested that changes in neural drive, recruitment pattern efficiency or selectivity, and inhibition of protective mechanisms may also be responsible. In summary, some studies have found that eccentric training is mode specific, improving only eccentric gains, while other studies have found improvements in both concentric and eccentric strength following eccentric training. Findings regarding functional performance and eccentric training are controversial. Factors responsible for the measured improvements are yet to be clarified.

f. Isokinetics and detection of training related changes in performance

Wilson and Murphy (1995) investigated the effectiveness of a battery of standard tests in detecting training related changes in functional sports performance. They assessed dynamic performance using the peak power output on a 6-second stationary cycle test. The assessment included the following: 1) maximum vertical jump height with a counter-movement, 2) isokinetic knee extension PT, and 3) maximum rate of isometric force development. Both isokinetic and vertical jump tests were significantly related to cycling performance both pre- and post-training, while the isometric test was related to cycling performance only pre-training. The isokinetic and vertical jump tests were also able to differentiate between individuals who were classified as poor, average or good cyclists, whereas the isometric test was unable to discriminate between the groups of performers. This was despite the isometric (static) test being done in a body position specific to the cycling action. The authors suggested that the observations may be attributable to neural differences between isometric and isokinetic (dynamic) modes of exercise. Differences in the activation patterns of isometric and dynamic muscle actions at the same joint angle have been demonstrated (Nakazawa et al 1993). The differing neural responses evoked by specific types of tests may explain the better correlation with dynamic than with static muscle tests. Further, when devising tests for predicting performance, the same neuro-mechanical characteristics must be employed.

2. Sport-specific talent identification

The identification of talent in athletic populations not only requires knowledge of the most desirable components of sports performance, but also appropriate and reliable ways of evaluating these qualities. The most discussed talent identification programs were employed in the former Eastern European countries, most notably East Germany. Currently, China has specialist sports schools in each of the provinces, and the American university system supports talented athletes (Figure 3-17). Many of the former Eastern European countries developed and adopted a systematic method of assessment and observation of school children by specialized physical education teachers. A variety of measures, such as height, weight, sprinting speed and endurance capacity, were taken, coupled with subjective measures, such as coordination and ball games skills. On the results, children were directed into broad categories of sport, for example those which require motor control, such as gymnastics (Figure 3-18), diving and ball games. Later, selected children would go to specialist schools, where continuous monitoring of physiological capabilities, psychological function, body shape and size, and skill development would ensure that time and effort was not spent on individuals without the necessary potential to excel in the chosen sport. Critical performance factors were assessed according to biological, not chronological age. Eventually, the outstanding athletes were sent to specialist sports schools and to the institutes of sport to be coached by the best professionals. Few have doubted the effectiveness of these programs in producing world class athletes, although the ethics have been questioned. In the West, nurturing of talent related to music, the arts and mathematics, for example, is often seen as a right, while to do the same with sporting talent is somehow seen as unethical.

Tanner, in the early 1960s, was the first to search for specific features in track and field athletes and weightlifters which could be associated with superior performance. He discovered that, to be successful in, for example, discus throwing, one needs to have long arms, relative to body height, and to be tall. The release of the discus then occurs at a higher point, offering a mechanical advantage and favoring the generation of greater angular velocity as the discus is

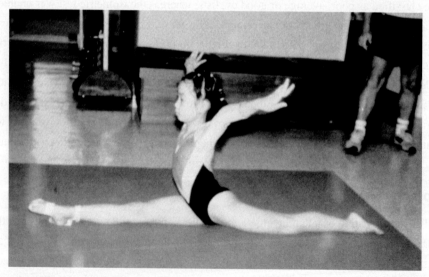

Figure 3-17 A young athlete during training.

released. In weightlifting, short limbs relative to body height are an advantage. The load is required to be moved through a shorter distance with lesser elevation of the center of gravity and less force is required to produce a lift with short levers. High-jumpers require long legs relative to body height, allowing clearance of bar height.

One way of determining the attributes which contribute to successful sports performance is to investigate differences between elite and non-elite performers. The relative importance of the differences found is then determined for each individual sport. Many physiological characteristics can be significantly improved by training. Yet, many characteristics have a genetically determined ceiling, which limits the scope for improvement. It is therefore important to examine these characteristics in relation to the individual's training background, ie, how much scope there is for further improvement.

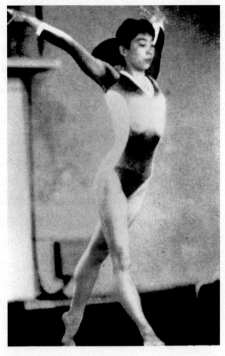

Figure 3-18 The actions of a gymnast require a high level of motor control.

3. Sport-specific profiling: a special reference to isokinetic strength testing

The evaluation of muscle strength and local muscular endurance are essential factors in sport-specific profiling. However, to obtain a comprehensive picture of the athletes strengths and weaknesses, cardiorespiratory, anthropometric, neurologic, flexibility, biochemistry and psychometric data will be needed (Komadel 1988). Such profiles can be used as a norm for a given sport, highlighting areas of physical fitness of particular relevance to the sport. The relative importance of the different aspects of fitness (strength, power, endurance, flexibility, body composition) and of necessary skills for a given sport may be elucidated by compiling profiles of successful performers in a single sport, and identifying the factors mainly responsible for their superior performance. Individual scores can be evaluated against norms for particular groups of athletes, allowing specific training recommendations to be made. Such data are also used to formulate selection criteria. To become an Olympic athlete requires both inherited and acquired characteristics. For example Klissouras (1971) studied the influence of heredity on VO_2max of monozygous twins. They found that the coefficient of heredity was extremely high (93.8). It is generally considered that there is a high genetic influence on speed, strength, power, coordination and balance, although this has not been proven (Komadel 1988). Longitudinal developmental studies are needed to evaluate the relative importance of heredity and training. Musculoskeletal profile data can also play an important role in the objective determination of specific rehabilitation goals and return-to-play criteria. It is important that such data are obtained only from athletes who have suffered no significant injury in the past, as this could be a confounding factor in subsequent measurements.

Muscle strength and endurance profiles, obtained by isokinetic testing, have been reported for a number of sports. Smith et al (1981) compared torque outputs of professional and elite (Olympic) amateur ice hockey players, in an attempt to evaluate the function of muscle groups important for performance. A higher shoulder abduction torque at slow speeds was found in the professional atheletes. This was regarded as both atttributable to the style of play, and indicative of capability of strong play, especially on the boards and in the corners. Sapega et al (1978) investigated sport-specific performance factors in Olympic fencers. They reported noticeable asymmetry of lower leg musculature. Moreover, fencers in different weapon categories demonstrated significant differences. Fencers were found to have outstanding leg strength and, despite an average of 26kg body mass difference, the swordsmen were nearly the equal of 1976 New York Jets football squad. Viitasalo et al (1981) investigated maximum isometric knee extension strength and various vertical jumping measures. They found that in contrast to the less well trained, isometric strength differences did not explain differences in performance in highly trained individuals. On the other hand, strengthening of the hip and/or the knee extensors has been reported as leading to improved vertical jump ability (Wiklander and Lysholm 1987, Tegner et al 1986). Anderson et al (1991) compared the relationships among isometric, isoinertial and isokinetic concentric and eccentric quadriceps and hamstring forces and the components of athletic performance, including vertical jump, 40-yard dash time and agility run time. The subjects were 39 male varsity athletes. The best predictor of 40-yard dash time was the right peak isokinetic concentric hamstring force at $60°/s$. The best predictor of the agility run time was the left mean isokinetic eccentric hamstring force at $90°/s$. Eccentric quadriceps and hamstring forces were not found to be better predictors of athletic performance than muscle force assessed in other ways. Hamiton et al (1992) studied the musculoskeletal characteristics of 28 elite professional ballet dancers and compared these to general population norms. In terms of isokinetically measured muscle strength, they reported that the men exhibited a striking imbalance between hip adbuctors (+18%) and adductors (-25%) when compared to the normal population. Weakness was found in the knee extensors (-16%) and flexors (-18%), but the extensor/flexor ratio was normal. Their ankle plantarflexors (+44%) and dorsiflexors (+40%) were significantly stronger than in the normal population. Again the strength ratio was normal. No significant bilateral differences were noted for the hip, knee and ankle strength. A similar reversal of strengths between hip/abductors (+21%) and adductors (-24%) was measured in women as in men. The women did not have the strength deficits about the knee found in men, their knee strength was normal, with a normal extension/flexion ratio. The strength in their ankles was even greater than that in the men for their size. Their plantarflexors (+33%) and dorsiflexors (+26%) were significantly above the norm, but the ratio was normal. A bilateral difference was found between right and left hip and knee strength: the right leg was stronger. On the whole, differences between elite ballet dancers and the general population were attributed to training and demands of corlograply, and to some extent, selection. In summary, isokinetic evaluation of muscle strength and endurance capacities can make a useful contribution to the development of sport-specific profiles of athletes. However, research in this field is still at its beginning.

SECTION 2

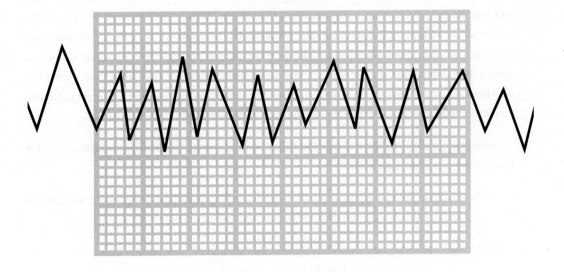

ISOKINETIC TECHNOLOGY:

A GLOBAL EXCHANGE

- Scientific Bases, Merits and Limitations -

IV. Round Table Discussion
A. Introduction by Tony Parker

In the past 30 years, isokinetic technology has been extensively researched in laboratories and practised in clinical and, to some extent, in sports settings. Section 1 has presented an overview of the scientific principles of isokinetic technology. Before presenting the section on practical applications of isokinetics, primarily based on the experience in the Asian setting, we would like to share the expert views and experiences of some of the world leading researchers and practitioners in this field. This section, "Global Exchange", aims to identify the specific merits and limitations of the practical use of isokinetics. The views of the individual author will be presented in a round table format allowing the readers to appreciate personal views and comparative arguments, and to make their own clinical judgment. Each individual expert has also been asked to highlight directions for future developments in research and practical applications in isokinetic science, thereby providing a stimulating forum for the readers.

Evidently, there is a global interest in the field of isokinetic technology to further develop the following scientific aspects:

1) Research on the validity and specificity of the different muscle actions such as eccentric actions, contraction, in relation to specific training and rehabilitation programs;

2) Identify the metabolic characteristics of and adaptations to isokinetic training;

3) Identify, simplify and validate sports-specific training programs;

4) Design user-friendly machines to bring the utilization of isokinetics closer to the sports field, and therefore, to cater for a wider market.

The crucial aspect of further development of isokinetic technology in the current health economy is to justify its usefulness and effectiveness in the overall patient care system, proving whether cost savings can be achieved with these appliances. Quantification of muscle performance provides objective data for the health care professional facilitating the design of an appropriate treatment program. This rational approach should be presented with the scientific support and clinical experience to the health care funding, health care policy makers and the health insurance industry. In order to survive in the current climate of health economics, the development of a new technology should strike a delicate balance between science and applicability. This section of "Global Exchange" is specifically directed toward evaluating this objective.

B. Todd S. Ellenbecker

1. Advantages of isokinetics

The use of isokinetics in orthopedic and sports physical therapy as a rehabilitative tool, as well as in the field of exercise physiology for performance enhancement and evaluation, has been extensively documented (Davies 1992). The continued publication of research highlighting the professional merits and applications of isokinetics as well as population specific normative data is imperative for the enhancement of this modality in both rehabilitation and sports training.

2. Isokinetics and manual muscle training

The relationship between manual muscle testing (MMT), the traditional form of muscular evaluation in clinical orthopedics, and isokinetics has been subjected to extensive investigations. Wilk and Andrews (1992) tested 175 consecutive patients following arthroscopic knee procedures with both MMT and isokinetic knee extension/flexion. All 175 patients had normal MMT scores for knee extension. The mean bilateral deficit with isokinetic testing of these patients with normal quadriceps strength concurred with MMT and it was 21% at 180°/s and 16% at 300°/s. Ellenbecker (1996) compared subjects with normal grade (5/5) MMT and isokinetic measurement of the shoulder internal and external rotators. Strength deficits ranging from 13% to 28% were found between extremities with isokinetic testing among subjects with normal grade manually assessed strength levels. These studies demonstrate the variability in muscular strength levels among individuals with normal MMT scores and provide rationale for the inclusion of isokinetic muscular strength evaluation particularly in individuals with normal grade muscle strength.

3. Isokinetic normative data

Another area of development in isokinetic application is the generation of normative data. While bilateral comparison of the injured to the uninjured extremity serves as a baseline clinical measurement, further interpretation of isokinetic testing can be accomplished via normative data normalized for body weight, as well as unilateral muscular strength ratios. Tables 4-1, 4-2 contain normative data samples from the Cybex isokinetic dynamometer regarding the muscular performance of elite junior tennis players generated in Scottsdale Sports Clinic, Arizona (Ellenbecker and Roetert 1995). Continued development of population and apparatus specific normative databases (Francis and Hoobler 1987) with large homogeneous subject populations will better allow clinicians and scientists to interpret isokinetic test variables.

4. Muscular endurance testing

Additional study of isokinetic variables not previously published will also serve to enhance

Motion (mean, °/s)	Dominant Arm		Nondominant Arm	
	Peak Torque (%) Body Weight	Work (%) Body Weight	Peak Torque (%) Body Weight	Work (%) Body Weight
External rotation				
Males, 210	12	20	11	19
Males, 300	10	18	10	17
Females, 210	8	14	8	15
Females, 300	8	11	7	12
Internal rotation				
Males, 210	17	32	14	27
Males, 300	15	28	13	23
Females, 210	12	23	11	19
Females, 300	11	15	10	13
External rotation: internal rotation ratio				
Males, 210	51	64	80	78
Males, 300	70	65	81	80
Females, 210	70	66	79	82
Females, 300	67	69	77	80

Rehabilitation of shoulder and elbow injures in tennis players.

Shoulder external and internal rotation isokinetic peak torque and single repetition work-to-body-weight ratios from 60 males and 38 females elite junior tennis players aged 12-17.

A Cybex 300 series isokinetic dynamometer and 90° of glenohumeral joint abduction were used. Data expressed in foot-pounds per unit of body weight.

Table 4-1 Isokinetic internal and external rotation strength in elite junior tennis players.

the clinical and scientific knowledge of the musculoskeletal system. One example is found in the application of endurance testing of the rotator cuff musculature. Previous endurance testing, popularized by Thorstensson (1976) for the lower extremities, has been successfully used for the upper extremity. Thirty-three elite junior tennis players performed twenty maximal concentric repetitions of internal and external rotation with 90° of glenohumeral joint abduction on a Cybex isokinetic dynamometer at 300°/s. Results of this testing showed statistically lower endurance ratios for the external rotators (65%) as compared to the internal rotators (82%). Further research on the endurance ratio in individuals with shoulder pathology is required to better understand the relationship between muscular endurance and injury.

Knee extension/flexion data for peak torque and single repetition work-to-body-weight ratios for elite junior male tennis players.

Variable/speed	Left		Right		t-value	Sig
	mean	S.D.	mean	S.D.		
Knee extension:						
Torque/BW 180	60.2	21.7	60.5	22.5	0.30	0.766
Torque/BW 300	53.8	6.8	54.0	8.8	0.22	0.827
Work/BW 180	61.4	23.5	62.1	24.5	0.47	0.644
Work/BW 300	54.1	12.7	52.8	12.6	1.72	0.090
Knee flexion:						
Torque/BW 180	36.6	13.5	36.0	13.5	1.04	0.305
Torque/BW 300	33.7	5.9	32.6	5.9	1.41	0.168
Work/BW 180	35.2	13.6	35.2	14.3	0.03	0.973
Work/BW 300	29.5	8.1	29.5	7.7	0.06	0.954

*All values expressed in foot-pounds relative to body weight in pounds.

Knee extension/flexion data for peak torque and single repetition work-to-body-weight ratios for elite junior female tennis players.

Variable/speed	Left		Right		t-value	Sig
	mean	S.D.	mean	S.D.		
knee extension:						
Torque/BW 300	44.4	5.5	47.4	6.7	2.31	0.049
Work/BW 300	43.3	7.6	42.6	7.2	0.60	0.554
Knee flexion:						
Torque/BW 330	30.7	6A	31.3	4.9	0.57	0.584
Work/BW 300	27.2	7.0	26.5	5.9	0.96	0.348

*All values expressed in foot-pounds relative to body weight in pounds.

Hamstring/quadricep peak torque ratio and single repetition work ratios for male and female junior tennis players.

Variable	Left		Right	
	Torque	Work	Torque	Work
Males:				
H/Q 180	61%	58%	59%	58%
H/Q 300	63%	55%	62%	56%
Females:				
H/Q 300	69%	64%	66%	63%

*All values expressed as percent hamstring strength relative to quadricep strength.

Table 4-2 Isokinetic normative data for knee extension/flexion strength in elite junior tennis players (65 males, 25 females).

This study does support the use of isokinetic exercise to improve local muscular endurance of the external rotators in tennis players, and highlights an inequality of endurance performance between the internal and external rotators in this population.

5. Open versus closed isokinetic testing

Isokinetic testing to assess lower extremity strength following ACL reconstruction has been extensively studied with isokinetic training and testing forming an integral part of many post-operative protocols. Recent emphasis on CKC training and testing in clinical orthopedics has changed many clinical rehabilitation programs by increasing the emphasis on the CKC environment (Bynum et al 1995).

Feiring and Ellenbecker (1995) tested 23 patients, after an average of 15-week period post-ACL reconstruction, using both a traditional OKC isokinetic knee extension/flexion movement, as well as an isokinetic CKC extension (leg press) movement. Results showed that the closed chain isokinetic peak torque and work on the injured limb was 92% to 95% of that measured in the uninjured limb. Open kinetic chain knee extension testing conducted at the same time revealed peak torque and work values of 71% to 75% of the uninjured limb. The results of this study demonstrate significant differences between open and closed chain muscle function 15 weeks after ACL reconstruction . The addition of muscular substitution and compensation made possible through the multiple, interconnecting segments in the CKC testing and training may explain the greater degree of symmetry in muscular strength in the lower extremities with the CKC testing in this study. Further research is needed to better understand the relationship between open and closed chain testing and training, in the rehabilitation of upper and lower extremity injuries.

6. Isokinetics and functional performance

As isokinetic technology and application improve in the future, a better understanding between muscular strength and functional performance will be developed. Several studies have found statistically significant correlations between isokinetic muscular strength testing and human performance. Feltner et al (1994) reported a decrease in rearfoot pronation following a period of 8-week of isokinetic inversion and eversion strengthening in runners. Pawlowski and Perrin (1989) found statistically significant correlations between shoulder internal and external rotation strength at 240 °/s and throwing velocity in collegiate baseball pitchers. Pedegana et al (1992) found a relationship between elbow and wrist extension and throwing velocity in professional baseball pitchers. Increases in serving velocity among elite tennis players were found following a 6-week period of isokinetic training of the internal and external rotators (Mont et al 1994, Ellenbecker et al 1988). Fleck et al (1992) reported a significant relationship between shoulder extension, horizontal adduction and internal rotation, as well as elbow extension/flexion strength and ball velocity in Olympic level team handball players. Finally, Roetert et al

(1996) found a significant relationship between isokinetic trunk extension/flexion strength and tennis specific medicine ball tosses in elite junior tennis players.

A better understanding of the relationship between functional activities and isokinetic exercise is necessary to optimally design and integrate isokinetic exercise in training programs to enhance performance and rehabilitate the human body. Further research profiling athletes and individuals with specific functional demands will assist clinicians and scientists with the interpretation of isokinetic test data. Continued progress in the technology of isokinetic dynamometers as well as research demonstrating the mechanical and physiological reliability of isokinetics will further the application of isokinetics to a broad spectrum of medical and scientific arenas.

References

1. Bynum EB, Barrack RL, Alexander AH. Open versus closed chain kinetic exercises after anterior cruciate ligament construction : A prospective randomized study. Am J Sports Med 23: 401-406, 1995.

2. Davies GJ. A Compendium of Isokinetics in Clinical Usage and Rehabilitation Techniques. 4th edition, 1992. La Crosse. WI, USA - S&S Publishers.

3. Ellenbecker TS. Muscular strength relationship between normal grade manual muscle testing and isokinetic measurement of the shoulder internal and external rotators. Submitted to Isokine Exerc Sci, 1996.

4. Ellenbecker TS, Roetert EP. Isokinetic muscular endurance of the rotator cuff in elite junior tennis players [Abs]. 1995. National Strength and Conditioning Association National Meeting, Phoenix, Arizona, USA.

5. Ellenbecker TS, Roetert EP. Concentric isokinetic quadricep and hamstring strength in elite junior tennis players. Isokine Exerc Sci 5: 3-6, 1995.

6. Eellenbecker TS, Davies GJ, Rowinski, MJ. Concentric versus eccentric isokinetic strengthening of the rotator cuff: Objective data versus functional test. Am J Sports Med 16: 64-69, 1988.

7. Feiring DC, Ellenbecker TS. Open versus closed chain testing with ACL reconstructed patients [Abs]. Med Sci Sports Exerc 27 (5): S106, 1995.

8. Feltner ME, Macrae HSH, Macrae PG. Strength training effects on rearfoot motion in running. Med Sci Sports Exerc 26: 1021-1027, 1994.

9. Fleck SJ, Smith SL, Craib MW, et al. Upper extremity isokinetic torque and throwing velocity in team handball. J Appl Sports Sci Res 6: 120-124, 1992.

10. Franics K , Hoobler T. Comparison of peak torque values of the knee flexor and extensor muscle groups using the Cybex II and Lido 2.0 isokinetic dynamometers. J Orthop Sports Phys Ther 8: 480-483, 1987.

11. Mont MA, Cohen DB, Campbell KR, et al. Isokinetic concentric versus eccentric training of shoulder rotators with functional evaluation of performance enhancement in elite tennis players. Am J Sports Med 22: 513-517, 1994.

12. Pawlowski D, Perrin DH. Relationship between shoulder and elbow isokinetic peak torque, torque acceleration energy, average power, and total work and throwing velocity in intercollegiate pitchers. Athletic Training 24: 129-132, 1989.

13. Pedegana LR, Elsner RC, Roberts D, et al. The relationship of upper extremity strength to throwing speed. Am J Sports Med 10: 352-354, 1992.

14. Roetert EP, McCormick TJ, Brown SW, Ellenbecker TS. Relationship between isokinetic and functionl trunk strength in elite junior tennis players. Isokine Exerc Sci accepted for publication, 1996.

15. Thorstensson A, Karlsson J. Fatiguability and fiber composition of human skeletal muscle. Acta Phys Scand, 98: 318-322, 1976

16. Wilk KE, Andrews JR. Comparison of normal grade manual muscle test to isokinetic testing of the knee extensors and flexors [Abs]. Phys Ther 1992.

C. Walter R. Frontera

1. The concept

Isokinetics is based on the concept that the angular velocity of a moving limb can be maintained constant by changing the force generated by a device to resist the intended movement. The force generated by a muscle is not constant throughout the range of motion, and depends on joint angle, bony leverage, and muscle fiber length-tension considerations. During an isokinetic movement, the device produces a force similar in magnitude to that produced by the muscle at every angle of the range of motion, but in the opposite direction. The limitation of isoinertial exercise training, ie, the resistance has to be matched with the weakest point of the range of motion, is therefore overcome.

Isokinetic movement is an artificial situation created in the research laboratory or in the clinic that does not exist in the natural environment nor in athletic competitions. These two situations are characterized by acceleration and deceleration of the moving limbs as well as variable levels of muscle force that are not matched by external resistances.

2. Measuring muscle strength

The need to quantify muscle strength in both the research laboratory and in the clinic cannot be overemphasized. For many years, clinicians in physical medicine and rehabilitation, orthopedics, and neurology depended on MMT to evaluate the strength of various muscle groups. These tests, although clinically useful in some conditions, lacked the sensitivity to detect minor but significant losses of muscle strength. Further, MMT was conducted under static conditions and usually at one or two joint angles. Great caution should be exercised when extrapolating these results to other joint angles and to dynamic conditions typical of everyday life activities and many athletic events.

In this regard, isokinetic devices have been shown to be very useful in evaluating muscle function. From my point of view, the advantages of isokinetic devices include the ability to test various muscle groups acting on different joints, the objective nature of the results, the capacity to evaluate different physiological characteristics of the muscle such as strength and endurance, the possibility of using visual feedback to motivate the subject, and the possibility of repeating the test under similar conditions to evaluate changes with training and/or rehabilitation.

3. Reliability

In the research laboratory as well as in the clinic, it is important to objectively quantify the changes in muscle strength that occur with interventions such as exercise training, immobilization, and/or rehabilitation. For a measurement to be useful, the inherent day-to-day variability of the test must be much smaller than the effects of the interventions. In other words, the method should be reliable. Good reliability is also necessary to achieve valid results. Muscle strength shows a relatively large variability between tests (reported values range between 5% and 20% under different conditions), which means that reliability of strength tests required special attention.

We have studied the reliability of an isokinetic dynamometer in 45- to 78-year-old men and women because of the increasing number of people in these age groups in many countries and the high prevalence of disability in this population. The strength of the knee and elbow extensors and flexors was tested twice under the same conditions at two different speeds 7 to 10 days apart. A significant correlation coefficient (Table 4-3) was found between the two tests at both speeds and in all muscle groups. However, there was a significant degree of variation between the coefficients. Also, we observed a statistically significant difference between the peak torques, with the second test always showing higher values in both sexes, speeds, and all muscle groups (Table 4-4). Our interpretation was that two tests may be needed to obtain a true peak torque in this population. We should keep this in mind, particularly in the clinic where practical limitations may not allow us to do a second test.

	Males	Females
60°/s		
KE	0.75	0.74
KF	0.70	0.62
EE	0.73	0.70
EF	0.84	0.78
240°/s or 180°/s		
KE	0.68	0.58
KF	0.77	0.66
EE	0.71	0.67
EF	0.77	0.72

*$p < 0.01$

Note : KE = knee extensor, KF = knee flexor, EE = elbow extensor, EF = elbow flexor.

Table 4-3 Pearson's correlation coefficients (r)* for two tests of isokinetic muscle strength in 45- to 78-year-old men and women. (Reproduced from Frontera et al. Arch Phys Med Rehabil 74: 1181, 1993.)

	Males 1	Males 2*	Females 1	Females 2*
KE				
60°/s	145	158	90	95
240°/s	83	90	48	54
KF				
60°/s	76	87	45	51
240°/s	45	54	28	31
EE				
60°/s	40	44	20	24
180°/s	30	32	14	16
EF				
60°/s	43	47	19	21
180°/s	30	33	13	14

*Second test significantly higher in both muscle groups and velocities.

Note : KE = knee extensor, KF = knee flexor, EE = elbow extensor, EF = elbow flexor.

Table 4-4 Mean peak torque (Nm) in two isokinetic strength tests of the dominant knee and elbow extensors and flexors in 45- to 78-year-old men and women. (Reproduced from Frontera et al. Arch Phys Med Rehabil 74: 1181, 1993.)

4. Limitations

There are certain factors that may limit the use of isokinetic devices and/or the interpretation of the collected data. Among them are the assumption that the angular velocity is truly constant, the anatomical and technical difficulties in testing some joints, the difficulties in isolating a single muscle group and stabilizing other body parts to limit the contribution of synergistic muscles, the lack of normative data for some patient populations and conditions, the lack of reliability and validation studies for some of the numerical values included in a typical report, and the cost of the equipment.

5. Specific applications in rehabilitation

Isokinetic devices have been used in rehabilitation for testing and training purposes. They are useful to objectively quantify the initial status of a patient and the progress made during rehabilitation. Also, it may be possible to estimate the extent of the neuromuscular deficit and to advise the patient on the required time for achieving a goal. If the test is repeated at different stages, it may also be possible to adjust the rehabilitation according to the findings, for example changing the exercise prescription if the desired gains have not been achieved. Finally, the strategies commonly used in the rehabilitation of various injuries and pathological states must be based on solid scientific research. In some cases, data to support our clinical approaches are lacking. Isokinetic devices may be useful research tools in a rehabilitation setting, and should be combined with other techniques to further our understanding of the neuromuscular adaptations resulting from the various rehabilitative strategies.

6. Future directions

To make isokinetics more useful and accessible, the limitations mentioned above must be addressed. In particular, the need for more research on the theoretical and practical aspects of isokinetics must be given high priority. Devices must be designed to respond to a large variety of clinical situations such as evaluations of athletes in the playing field. This would require portable and less expensive devices. Such devices may also be of benefit in the clinic when a large number of patients or athletes are to be screened. The addition of eccentric testing must be further developed, since research studies have demonstrated the importance of this type of muscle action for the development of strength. Finally, health professionals in Sports Medicine and Rehabilitation should be educated on the benefits and limitations of isokinetics.

References

1. Frontera WR, Hughes VA, Evans WJ. Reliability of isokinetic muscle strength testing in 45- to 78-year-old men and women. Arch Phys Med Rehabil 74: 1181-1185, 1993.

D. Scott M. Lephart and Danny M. Pincivero

Isokinetic dynamometry has evolved considerably since its inception by Hislop and Perrine in 1967. The ability to objectively quantify and document muscular strength has given Sports Medicine clinicians and researchers the opportunity to greatly expand the current body of knowledge. By fixing the angular velocity of movement through accommodating resistance, isokinetic dynamometry allows isolated muscle groups to exert maximal force throughout the full range of motion. This unique feature has allowed objective comparisons between limbs as well as between agonist and antagonist muscle groups. These measurements have resulted in the generation of various bilateral and reciprocal muscle group ratios among the general and athletic populations. Researchers and clinicians alike have benefited from such information in comparing individuals experiencing musculoskeletal pathology.

The objectivity offered by isokinetic dynamometry, however, loses its application when compared to functional activities. To date, most isokinetic dynamometers do not exceed angular velocities of 450°/s. This test velocity pales in comparison to motions such as baseball pitching, where the angular velocity of the glenohumeral joint often exceeds 5,000°/s (Perrin 1993). In addition, it is difficult to equate the constant velocity movement of the isokinetic dynamometer with the more ballistic functional activities. The inability of isokinetics to detect joint acceleration and deceleration throughout functional speeds remains a major limitation.

Another major concern in the literature is the relationship between contraction speeds and muscle fiber types. It has been suggested that variations in the order of motor unit recruitment are likely to be dictated by the angular velocity of the test protocol (Perrin 1993). However, it has been shown, at the higher test velocities, that the recruitment of fast twitch (FT) fibers predominates in order to allow the joint to match the preset angular velocity of the dynamometer (Suter et al 1993, Coyle et al 1981, Gregor et al 1979). Based on the notion that slow twitch (ST) fibers are recruited first, followed by FT fibers as the magnitude and duration of tension increases, it would appear that maximal or near maximal recruitment of both ST and FT fibers would occur independently of the various angular velocities (Perrin 1993, Sherman et al 1982). Further research is required to investigate the relationship between muscle fiber type recruitment patterns, test velocity and test protocol.

1. Modalities for strength assessment and development

Isokinetic exercise and assessment can be considered as one of the most objective measures of muscular strength. Although the strength of a muscle group can be measured by other modes of exercise (namely, isometric and isoinertial), these methods lack the objective generation of values such as peak torque, work and power that isokinetic dynamometry provides. Furthermore, most isokinetic dynamometers have the capability to provide objective measures of isometric strength at various angles in the range of motion. Once again, the major limitation is the applicability of isokinetic-derived results to functional activities (ie, closed kinetic chain). Isolated quadriceps and hamstring contraction at a constant velocity do not appear to approximate the co-contraction nature of closed kinetic chain activities. If the objective of the research question or rehabilitation protocol is to isolate and evaluate a particular muscle group, isokinetic exercise may be the modality of choice. It should be kept in mind, however, that some cautions should be warranted when attempting to apply a direct relationship between a lower extremity open kinetic chain isokinetic evaluation and closed kinetic chain functional activities.

2. Application to Sports Medicine

Within the field of Sports Medicine, isokinetic exercises have been successfully utilized and documented both in the research and clinical settings. Although an accurate isokinetic evaluation can give valuable information on specific muscle groups, it must be remembered that it is limited to this function. Attempting to quantify an individual's sports performance and functional ability based on an isokinetic evaluation would be inappropriate (Perrin 1993). However, the application of isokinetic exercise to injury rehabilitation can be significant. In addition, isokinetic evaluations may be able to detect bilateral or reciprocal muscle group imbalances which may be related to various musculoskeletal overuse disorders in the physically active individual. The ability to identify bilateral or reciprocal muscle group imbalances allows isokinetics to be used as a screening device prior to the commencement of physical activity which, in many cases, may precede musculoskeletal pathology. It should be noted, however, that bilateral asymmetry in individuals such as baseball players may be observed from an isokinetic evaluation. Athletes participating in sports that require symmetrical body motions should display fewer bilateral muscle group differences (Perrin 1993). An isokinetic evaluation can also be used as a tool for the assessment of training-induced changes in major muscle groups, although the specificity of the activity must be considered.

3. Future directions

The role of isokinetics as a reliable modality for the measurement of muscular function has received adequate attention in the literature concerning commonly used testing protocols. More sport-specific and functional patterns of movement need to be investigated in greater depth regarding the efficacy of such protocols (eg, PNF diagonal patterns mimicking throwing motion). The reliability and validity of isokinetic muscular endurance protocols is another area that should be considered for future research. A major question that often arises is whether or not a relationship exists between velocity of movement and duration of protocol with differential muscle fiber metabolism (ST versus FT). The ability to quantify the metabolic characteristics of different muscle fibers in response to varying isokinetic speeds and durations would allow future research to address the issue of specificity of training with activity.

References

1. Coyle EF, Feiring DC, Rotkis TC, Cote III RW, Roby FB, Lee W, Wilmore JH. Specificity of power improvements through slow and fast isokinetic training. J Appl Physiol: Respirat Environ Exerc Physiol 51(6): 1437-1442, 1981.

2. Gregor RJ, Edgerton VR, Perrine JJ, Campion DS, DeBus C. Torque-velocity relationships and muscle fiber composition in elite female athletes. J Appl Physiol: Respirat, Environ, Exerc Physiol 47 (2): 338-392, 1979.

3. Hislop HJ, Perrine JJ. The isokinetic concept of exercise. Phys Ther 47 (2): 114-117, 1967.

4. Perrin DH. Isokinetic Exercise and Assessment, 1993. Human Kinetics Publishers. Champaign, IL.

5. Sherman WM, Pearson DR, Plyley MJ, Costill DL, Habansky AJ, Vogelgesang DA. Isokinetic rehabilitation after surgery. Am J Sport Med 10: 155-161, 1982.

6. Suter E, Herzog W, Sokolosky J, Wiley JP, Macintosh BR. Muscle fiber type distribution as estimated by Cybex testing and by muscle biopsy. Med Sci Sport Exerc 25: 363-370, 1993.

E. Terry R. Malone and William E. Garrett

The utilization of clinical isokinetics has become nearly ubiquitous in the measurement of strength. Dynamometers have evolved to allow high velocity and high torque as well as the assessment of concentric and eccentric muscle action. Although some individuals argue the testing velocity is limited (450°/s to 500°/s), these values are assessed in a "closed" environment allowing rotation about a single axis and requiring relatively pure rotational assessment (torque). It must be noted that isokinetics allows us to assess the neural system's ability to maximally activate and drive the musculature in an isolated form. The high velocities that are achieved in throwing and kicking involve the utilization of the limb as a whip and allow the accumulation of multiple segments providing very high velocities through multiple joints. When a segment becomes isolated and rotation about a single axis is controlled (as in single axis dynamometer), the ability to generate high velocities is greatly minimized. A second limitation of open chain assessment has been the description of lack of "functionality" related to both action (isolated versus integrated muscle utilization) and velocity (both terminal and mainte-nance of a specific velocity that has been pre-selected). The first portion of this limitation is both a strength and a limitation. The strength being that it allows us to determine how an iso-lated muscle group is activated, but that is also a weakness as it does not tell us how well it is integrated in the normal recruitment process. While velocity control is provided by dynamometry, patients do accelerate to the pre-selected maximal velocity and decelerate from it much as they do in typical functional activities. This is not to say that it is a replication of absolute functional patterns but does provide one form of assessment of a particular pattern. Interestingly, concentric isokinetic assessment has typically shown a high correlation to func-tional tests.

Recognition of the importance of the eccentric activation has provided a stimulus for the incorporation of this measurement into our total assessment of the individual patient. We have found that concentric assessment is more consistent but eccentric assessment does provide addi-tional information regarding the ability of an individual to use multiple demand of neuromuscular patterns in a meaningful way. It has been our experience that the integration of eccentric activities through a CPM sequence on the isokinetic dynamometer seems to be very readily accepted by the patient and can then be followed at a later time by the active eccentric action requiring a higher level of neural integration. The last facet of eccentric integration is to use the stretch-shortening cycle of function primarily through depth jumping, hopping, multiple jumping tasks, and lunging activities in an integrated functional pattern.

There is no question that the use of isokinetics allows us to quantify to a much higher level of the neural system's ability to drive individual muscle groups. This assessment is quite useful in determining the individual's readiness and ability to request muscular activation. Isolated OKC assessment will demonstrate a very significant alteration in performance when compared with a CKC multiple joint integrated pattern. Thus, it is very important not to allow larger muscle groups to substitute for "involved" groups, which may be the case in allowing lower extremity functional activities when significant muscle inhibition or lack of the ability for normal recruitment is present.

1. Strength assessment and applications to Sports Medicine

The objectivity provided through clinical assessment using isokinetic dynamometry is no longer in question. Although a direct application of OKC single joint assessment is not appropriate, it has been shown to have a very strong correlation and predictive value and does allow us to more fully elucidate the weak link in any musculoskeletal chain. As we have always believed in integrated assessments, it would be our recommendation that open chain and closed chain activities continue to be utilized in that format rather than allowing them to stand alone. This is particularly true in the sports environment where the more numerous the demands that can be placed on the neuromuscular system, the more likely the system is to be responsive to a specific demand at any point in time. The neuromuscular response or neurophysiologic action may not be exactly the same for an eccentric activation through the CPM mode, the active mode (machine eccentric), or the stretch-shortening cycle, yet the more varied the request for activity the greater the likelihood of an appropriate response when faced with such in an athletic endeavor. Hence, we recommend integrating multiple activities and emphasize the importance of assessment being performed in the same way. It must also be recognized that the assessment must be performed on a clinically silent joint as any pain or effusion will greatly alter the individual's ability to produce maximal effort. Although maximal efforts are ideal in training, frequently sub-maximal activities which can be provided through isokinetic dynamometry are very useful for endurance and safe applications of specific doses for exercise demands (Garrett and Malone, AAOS Instructional Course Lectures 1993). Too often assessments are made on an inhibited structure, thus providing inappropriate and non-useful information. It is our belief that isokinetics will be more greatly integrated into different applications to sports through creative applications of both open and closed patterns in a speed controlled environment.

2. Future directions

Many concepts have been presented previously regarding greater integration rather than isolation of isokinetics in the aforementioned paragraphs. Unfortunately, many clinicians have been led to believe that the use of isokinetics is not appropriate in an isolated OCK format. The medical community should recognize that properly applied isokinetic assessment in an OKC does provide significant information regarding the neural system's ability to drive the muscular system in a somewhat isolated environment. This information is very useful and provides comparisons between limbs as well as comparisons to normative values for body weight. It will help future applications which will also allow comparisons based on individual muscle composition (glycolytic versus oxidative) and possible greater predictive values of muscular performance. The application of isokinetics to the trunk is quite exciting as spectral analysis has been coupled to isokinetic assessment and fatigue assessment as well as other performance variables which are increasingly available to clinicians. Additional integration of electromyography technology to OKC and CKC integrated isokinetic devices will be welcomed by future clinicians. The application/integration of joint position sense dynamometric assessment is also quite exciting. We may find that the use of CKC isokinetics will allow excellent exercise activity, but may not be as useful as an evaluation tool.

Further Readings

1. Anderson MA, Gieck JH, Perrin D, Weltman A, Ruth R, Denegar C. The relationship among isometric, isotonic and isokinetic concentric and eccentric quadriceps and hamstring force and three components of athletic performance. J Orthop Sports Phys Ther 14: 114-120, 1991.

2. Brask B, Lueke RH, Soderberg GL. Electromyographical analysis of selected muscles during the lateral step-up exercise. Phys Ther 64: 324-329, 1984.

3. Bunton EE, Pitnez WA, Kane AW, Cappnert TA. The role of limb torque, muscle action and proprioception during closed kinetic chain rehabilitation of the lower extremity. J Athletic Training 28: 10-20, 1993.

4. Chandler TJ, Wilson GD, Store MH. The Effects of the Squat Exercise on Knee Stability. Med Sci Sports Exerc 21: 299-303, 1989.

5. Davies GJ. A Compendium of Isokinetics in Clinical Usage and Rehabilitation Techniques, 4th edition, 1992. WI S & S Publishers, Onalaska.

6. DeCarlo M, Porter DA, Gehlsen G, Bahamonde R. Electromyographic and cinematographic analysis of the lower extremity during closed and open kinetic chain exercise. Isokine Exerc Sci 2: 24-29, 1992.

7. DeNuccio DK, Davies GJ, Rowinski MJ. Comparison of quadriceps isokinetic eccentric and isokinetic concentric data using a standard fatigue protocol. Isokine Exerc Sci 1: 81-86, 1991.

8. Draganich LF, Jaeger RJ, Kralj AR. Coactivation of the hamstrings and quadriceps during extension of the knee. J Bone Joint Surg 71(A): 1075-1081, 1989.

9. Draganich LF, Vahey JW. An in vitro study of anterior cruciate ligament strain induced by quadriceps and hamstring forces. J Orthop Res 8: 57-63, 1990.

10. Garrett WE, Malone TR. The modality of therapeutic exercise: Instructional Course Lecturers. Am Acad Orthop Surg 42: 453-459, 1993.

11. Gleim GW, Nicholas JA, Webb JN. Isokinetic evaluation following leg injuries. Phys Sportsmed 6: 74-82, 1978.

12. Graham VL, Gehlsen GM, Edwards JA. Electromyographic evaluation of closed and open kinetic chain knee rehabilitation exercises. J Athletic Training 28: 23-30, 1993.

13. Gryzlo SM, Patek RM, Pink M, Perry J. Electromyographic analysis of knee rehabilitation exercises. J Orthop Sports Phys Ther 20: 36-43, 1994.

14. Harter RA, Osternig LR, Singer KM, James SL, Larson RL, Jones DC. Long-term evaluation of knee stability and function following surgical reconstruction for anterior cruciate ligament insufficiency. Am J Sports Med 16: 434-443, 1988.

15. Howell SM. Anterior tibial translation during a maximum quadriceps contraction: Is it clinically significant? Am J Sports Med 18: 573-578, 1990.

16. Lephart SM, et al. Functional assessment of the anterior cruciate insufficient knee [Abs]. Med Sci Sports Exerc 20: 2, 1988.

17. Lephart SM, Perrin DH, Fu FH, Minger K. Functional performance tests for the anterior cruciate ligament insufficient athlete. J Athletic Training 26: 44-50, 1991.

18. Lutz GE, Palmitier RA, An KN, Chao EYS. Comparison of tibiofemoral joint forces during open kinetic chain and closed kinetic chain exercises. J Bone Joint Surg Am 75(A): 732-739, 1993.

19. Lutz GE, Palmitier RA, An KN, Chao EYS. Closed kinetic chain exercises for athletes after reconstruction of the anterior cruciate ligament [Abs]. Med Sci Sports Exerc 23: 413, 1991.

20. Markolf KL, Bargar WL, Shoemaker SC, Amstutz HC. Role of joint load in knee stability. J Bone Joint Surg 63(A): 579-585, 1981.

21. Markolf KL, Kochan A, Amstutz HC. Measurement of knee stiffness and laxity in patients with documented absence of anterior cruciate ligament. J Bone Joint Surg 66(A) : 242-253, 1984.

22. Markolf KL, Gorek JF, Kabo JM, Shapiro MS. Direct measurement of resultant forces in the anterior cruciate ligament. J Bone Joint Surg 72(A): 557-567, 1990.

23. Palmitier RA, An KN, Scott SG, Chao EYS. Kinetic chain exercise in knee rehabilitation. Sports Med 11: 402-413, 1991.

24. Renström P, Arms SW, Stanwyck TS, Johnson RJ, Pope MH. Strain within the anterior cruciate ligament during hamstring and quadriceps activity. Am J Sports Med 14: 83-87, 1986.

25. Reynolds NL, Worrell TW, Perrin DH. Effect of a lateral step-up exercise protocol on quadriceps isokinetic peak torque values and thigh girth. J Orthop Sports Phys Ther 15: 151-155, 1992.

26. Robertson DGE, Fleming D. Kinetics of standing broad and vertical jumping. Can J Sports Sci 12: 19-23, 1987.

27. Shoemaker SC, Markolf KL. Effects of joint load on the stiffness and laxity of ligament-deficient knees. J Bone Joint Surg Am 67(A): 136-146, 1985.

28. Tegner Y, Lysholm J, Lysholm M, Gillquist J. A performance test to monitor rehabilitation and evaluate anterior cruciate ligament injuries. Am J Sports Med 14: 156-159, 1986.

29. Timm KE: Post-surgical knee rehabilitation: A 5-year study of four methods and 5,381 patients. Am J Sports Med 16: 463-468, 1988.

30. Wilk KE, et al. The relationship between subjective knee scores, isokinetic testing, and functional testing in the ACL reconstructed knee. J Orthop Sports Phys Ther 20: 60-73, 1994.

31. Wilk KE, Andrews JR. The effects of pad placement and angular velocity on tibial displacement during isokinetic exercise. J Orthop Sports Phys Ther 17: 23-30, 1993.

32. Whieldon T, Yack J, Collins C. Anterior tibial displacement during weight bearing and non-weight bearing rehabilitation exercises in the anterior cruciate deficient knee [Abs]. Phys Ther 69: 151, 1989.

33. Wyatt MP, Edwards AM. Comparison of quadriceps and hamstring torque values during isokinetic exercise. J Orthop Sports Phys Ther 3: 48-56, 1981.

34. Yack HJ, Collins CE, Whieldon TJ. Comparison of closed and open kinetic chain exercise in the anterior cruciate ligament deficient knee. Am J Sports Med 21: 49-54, 1993.

Further Readings on Shoulder

1. Guanche C, Knatt T, Solomonow M, Lu Y, Baratta R. The synergistic action of the capsule and the shoulder muscles. Am J Sports Med 23(3): 301-306, 1995.

2. Lephart SM, Warner JP, Borsa PA, Fu FH. Proprioception of the shoulder joint in healthy, unstable and surgically repaired shoulders. J Shoulder Elbow Surg 3(6): 371-380, 1994.

3. O'Brien SJ, Neves MC, Arnoczky SP, Rozbruck SR, DiCarlo EF, Warren RF, Schwartz R, Wickiewicz TL. The anatomy and histology of the inferior glenohumeral ligament complex of the shoulder. Am J Sports Med 18(5): 449-456, 1990.

4. Sharkey NA, Marder RA. The rotator cuff opposes superior translation of the humeral head. Am J Sports Med 23(3): 270-275, 1995.

5. Smith RL, Brunolli J. Shoulder kinesthesia after glenohumeral joint dislocation. Phys Ther 69: 106-112, 1989.

6. Speer KP, Xianghua D, Torzilli PA, Altchek DA, Warren RF. Strategies for ran anterior capsular shift of the shoulder: A biomechanical comparison. Am J Sports Med 23(3): 264-269, 1995.

F. Christer G. Rolf

Since the presentation of the isokinetic method (Hislop and Perrine 1967), numerous studies have focused on single maximal concentric and, to minor extent, eccentric contractions (Westblad 1995 and references cited herein). The majority of investigations in the literature deal with knee extensor performance, which is also addressed in this section. Plantarflexors (Johansson and Gerdle 1988) and shoulder muscles (Wredmark et al 1992, Tsai et al 1991, Gerdle et al 1988) are also frequently tested. The purpose of this section is to address the question of what the isokinetic method really measures, and to critically discuss the reliability, validity and clinical implications of the method.

It may be argued that any measure of muscle performance should be related to well established physiological characteristics such as muscle fiber composition, muscle cross-sectional area and metabolic function. Isokinetic concentric knee extensor performance reflects the structural properties of the knee extensor muscles (Johansson 1987, Thorstensson 1976). Peak torques and contraction work are the most frequently used measures of isokinetic muscle output, often in combination with registration of electromyographic activity (Engström et al 1992, Elmqvist et al 1989, 1988, Gerdle et al 1988). Single contraction peak torque and contraction work were significantly correlated to the cross-sectional area of the vastus lateralis and to the type II fiber content of the muscle (Johansson et al 1987). Electromyographic measures indicated that the vastus lateralis was representative of the whole of the quadriceps muscle group in this essence. Considering isokinetic concentric knee extensor endurance, an arbitrary measure of contraction work and electromyographic activity was found to correlate with maximal oxygen uptake (VO_2max) in marathon runners (Lorentzon et al 1988). One may conclude that there is some basic scientific knowledge regarding structural and metabolic factors reflected by single as well as repetitive maximal concentric isokinetic measures.

Basic studies are required to improve the validity of the isokinetic method when used in clinical practice (Winter et al 1981). In a training follow-up study of orienteers, an increase in isokinetic knee extensor endurance was observed in parallel with an increase in running capacity at the anaerobic threshold (Johansson et al 1988, Sjödin and Jacobs 1981). In ice hockey players, the isokinetic endurance pattern changed non-systematically with training and games over a 2-year period (Johansson et al 1989). From a coaching perspective, it is of great importance if the isokinetic measures of isolated muscle groups reflect an individual's ability to perform functional movements (Sapega 1990, Mayhew and Rothstein 1985). The literature is divided regarding this issue. Knee torque measurements did not adequately characterize knee function in patients with various disorders (Krebs 1989, Lankhorst et al 1985). Low correlations were found between vertical jump ability and knee extensor concentric torque (Genuario and Dolgener 1980), in contrast with Bosco et al (1983). In the field of athletic performance, rehabilitation and injury prevention, objective measures of muscle function are essential. It must, however, be stressed that laboratory measurements do not necessarily reflect functional performance. Despite the wide clinical use of isokinetics, few studies of reliability, validity and clinical outcome have been performed (Mayhew and Rothstein 1985). Numerous questions may be raised on this issue from the clinicians' perspective regarding the gradual move toward earlier eccentric training in rehabilitation from injuries. It has been argued that muscle weakness or imbalance increases the risk of sustaining an overuse injury (Rolf 1995, Renström 1994, van Mechelen 1992, Taimela et al 1990). The importance of lower extremity eccentric muscle action in decelerating the body during walking and running is well recognized (Stauber 1989). The eccentric isokinetic mode has not been studied as much as the concentric (Westblad 1995, Westing et al 1990). What are then the structural, neuromuscular or metabolic bases for eccentric muscle performance measured by isokinetic methods? No definite answers are available, and future studies on isokinetics may well be focused here. There are several reasons why reproducible and valid methods for objective evaluation of eccentric muscle function, and endurance in particular, should be of interest.

1. Specific application

Isokinetic eccentric knee extensor muscle endurance has not been studied extensively. There are several clinical applications to be addressed. Excessive eccentric loading results in delayed muscle soreness (Fridén et al 1983). On the other hand, intracellular muscle damage is markedly reduced after eccentric training (Komi and Buskirk 1972). The fact that isokinetics is limited to quantification of isolated muscle performance may be regarded as a disadvantage, in particular when discussing eccentric contractions. Walking, running and jumping exploit the lower extremity kinetic chain, in which the muscles are activated synchronously during weight bearing (Palmitier et al 1991). It may consequently be argued that lower extremity eccentric muscle function should be studied in functionally more relevant movements such as walking and jumping (Rolf et al unpublished data). The muscles of the lower extremity are able to damp impact by a smooth force increase with simultaneous joint motion. It remains to be shown whether isokinetic eccentric measures reflect this functional capacity. Deficiencies in eccentric muscle performance may hypothetically cause a redistribution of loads to other muscle groups or passive structures during extensive loading (Johansson 1992, Stanish 1989, Rolf et al unpublished data). Patients with ACL-deficient knees showed a decreased eccentric relative to concentric knee extensor performance at a 5-year follow-up (Engström et al 1992). Whether this reflects insufficient rehabilitation or an inability to use the injured leg properly in daily activities remains to be solved. Eccentric contractions produce increased generation of force at reduced oxygen cost and perceived exertion compared with concentric contractions (Dean 1988). Mechanical efficacy increases with an increase in velocity of motion in contrast with concentric performance. At foot strike in running and jumping, the quadriceps muscles may stabilize the hip and knee joints. The elastic components of muscle may be of interest for performance and injury prevention, as at the end of a marathon race, the recoil characteristics of the muscle have deteriorated (Nicol et al 1991).

How can we measure eccentric endurance? A high reliability was found in one hundred consecutive maximal eccentric knee extensor actions at $90°/s$ in a test-re-test study on untrained volunteers, recording work and absolute endurance (Westblad and Johansson 1993). Eccentric strength studies require larger sample sizes than concentric ones. The question may be raised: what does eccentric "endurance" reflect in sports practice? The same experiment indicated a close relationship between total work during eccentric knee extensors and running economy in elite middle distance runners (Westblad et al 1996). One may hypothesize that this, to some extent, reflects the elastic components of the muscle. If this is true, could isokinetics be used to discriminate between athletes who are exposed to repetitive loading daily, being at risk of sustaining overuse injuries (Rolf 1995)? In trained ballet dancers, who are exposed to several hours of repetitive loading per day, an increased eccentric/concentric ratio of muscle endurance and also a higher absolute endurance were found compared to untrained controls (Westblad et al 1995). If this reflects a functional adaptation, one may speculate that a low ratio could be associated with an increased risk of overuse injuries, or indicate insufficient rehabilitation (Engström et al 1992).

2. Future developments

As discussed above, there are several topics to be addressed in the future. Let me speculatively address three major areas of interest. 1) From the biomechanical and physiological point of view, one implementation would be to study the role of isokinetic measures in a comprehensive in vivo approach considering functional movements, including measurements of internal and external forces and EMG as well as joint motion. 2) From a sports practice and physiotherapy perspective, there is a great need of sport-specific tests and validity studies on rehabilitation procedures. A consensus on reliable and valid isokinetic measures is essential. Power analyses should be conducted prior to all clinical studies in order to be able to draw relevant conclusions. Training studies comparing open versus closed chain actions may also be partly evaluated by isokinetic measures. 3) Finally, and perhaps most challenging for the clinicians, are studies on eccentric muscle performance in relation to the etiology and rehabilitation of overuse injury in sports.

References

1. Bosco C, Mognoni P, Luhtanen P. Relationship between isokinetic performance and ballistic movement. Eur J Appl Physiol 51: 357-364, 1983.

2. Dean E. Physiology and therapeutic implications of negative work. Phys Ther 68: 233-237, 1988.

3. Elmqvist L, Lorentzon R, Johansson C*, Fugl-Meyer A. Does a torn anterior cruciate ligament lead to change in the central nervous drive of the knee extensors? Eur J Appl Physiol 58: 203-207, 1988.

4. Elmqvist L, Lorentzon R, Johansson C*, Långström M, Fagerlund M, Fugl-Meyer A. Knee extensor muscle function before and after reconstruction of anterior cruciate ligament tear. Scand J Rehabil Med 21: 131-139, 1989.

5. Engström B, Westblad P, Johansson C*. Decreased eccentric muscle endurance in the conservatively treated anterior cruciate deficient knee. Scand J Med Sci Sports 2: 224-248, 1992.

6. Fridén J, Sjöström M, Ekblom B. Myofibrillar damage following intense eccentric exercise in man. Int J Sports Med 4: 170-176, 1983.

7. Genuario S, Dolgener F. The relationship of isokinetic torque at two speeds to vertical jump. Res Q 51: 593-598, 1980.

8. Gerdle B, Johansson C*, Lorentzon R. Relationships between work and electromyographic activity during repeated leg muscle contractions in orienteers. Eur J Appl Physiol 58: 8-12, 1988.

9. Hislop H, Perrine J. The isokinetic concept of exercise. Phys Ther 47: 114-117, 1967.

10. Johansson C*. Knee extensor performance in runners: Differences between specific athletes and implications for injury prevention. Sports Med 14: 75-81, 1992.

11. Johansson C*. Elite sprinters, ice hockey players, orienteers and marathon runners: Isokinetic leg muscle performance in relation to muscle structure and training. Thesis 1987. Umeå University. ISSN 0346-6612.

12. Johansson C*, Gerdle B. Mechanical output and IEMG of single and repeated isokinetic plantarflexions: A study of untrained and endurance trained women. Int J Sports Med 9: 330-333, 1988.

13. Johansson C*, Gerdle B, Lorentzon R, Rasmusson S, Reiz S, Fugl-Meyer A. Fatigue and endurance of lower extremity muscles in relation to running velocity at OBLA in male orienteers. Acta Physiol Scand 131: 203-209, 1988.

14. Johansson C*, Lorentzon R, Fugl-Meyer A. Isokinetic muscular performance in m quadriceps of elite ice hockey players. Am J Sports Med 1: 30-34, 1989.

15. Johasson C*, Lorentzon R, Rasmusson S, Reiz S, Haggmark S, Nyman H, Fugl-Meyer A. Peak torque and OBLA running capacity in male orienteers. Acta Physiol Scand 132: 525-530, 1988.

16. Johansson C*, Lorentzon R, Sjöström M, Fagerlund M, Fugl-Meyer A. Sprinters and marathon runners: Does isokinetic knee extensor performance reflect muscle size and structure? Acta Physiol Scand 130: 663-669,1987.

17. Komi P, Buskirk E. Effect of eccentric and concentric muscle conditioning on tension and electrical activity of human muscle. Ergonomics 15: 417-434, 1972.

18. Krebs D. Isokinetic, electrophysiologic and clinical function relationships following torniquet aided knee arthrotomy. Phys Ther 69: 803-815, 1989.

19. Lankhorst G, van der Stadt R, van der Korst J. The relationships of functional capacity, pain and isometric and isokinetic torque in osteoarthrosis of the knee. Scand J Rehabil Med 17: 167-172, 1985.

20. Lorentzon R, Johansson C*, Sjöström M, Fugl-Meyer A. Fatigue during dynamic contractions in male sprinters and marathon runners. Acta Physiol Scand 132: 531-536, 1988.

21. Mayhew T, Rothstein J. Measurement of muscle performance with instruments. In Rothstein JM Ed Measurement in Physical Therapy 57-102, 1985. Churchill Livingstone, New York.

22. Nicol C, Komi P, Marconnet P. Fatigue effects of marathon running on neuromuscular performance. I: Changes in muscle force and stiffness characteristics. Scand J Med Sci Sports 1: 10-17, 1991.

23. Palmitier R, An K, Scott S, Chao E. Kinetic chain exercise in knee rehabilitation. Sports Med 11: 402-413, 1991.

24. Renström P. An introduction to overuse injuries. In Harries M, Williams C, Stanish W, Micheli L. (Ed) Oxford Textbook of Sports Medicine 531-545, 1994. Oxford University Press.

25. Rolf C. Overuse injuries of the lower extremity in runners. Scand J Med Sci Sports 5: 181-190, 1995.

26. Rolf C, Westblad P, Ekenman I, Lundberg A, Murphy N, Lamontagne M, Halvorsen K. An experimental in vivo method for analysis of local deformation on tibial with simultaneous measures of ground reaction forces, forces on the tibia, lower extremity muscle activity and joint motion. Unpublished data, submitted for publication.

27. Sapega A. Muscle performance evaluation in orthopedic practice. J Bone Joint Surg Am 72: 1562-1574, 1990.

28. Sjödin B, Jacobs I. Onset of blood lactate accumulation and marathon running performance. Int J Sports Med 2: 23-26, 1981.

29. Stanish W. Overuse injuries in athletes: A perspective. Med Sci Sports Exerc 16: 1-7, 1989.

30. Stauber W. Eccentric action of muscles: Physiology, injury and adaptation. Exerc Sports Sci Rev 19: 157-185, 1989.

31. Taimela S, Kujala U, Osterman K. Intrinsic risk factors and athletic injuries. Sports Med 9: 205-215, 1990.

32. Thorstensson A. Muscle strength, fiber types and enzyme activities in man. Acta Physiol Scand Suppl 443, 1976.

33. Tsai L, Wredmark T, Johansson C*, Gibo K, Engström B, Törnqvist H. Shoulder function in patients with non-operated anterior shoulder instability. Am J Sports Med 5: 469-473, 1991.

34. van Mechelen W. Running injuries: A review of the epidemiological literature. Sports Med 14: 320-335, 1992.

35. Westblad P. On methods of evaluation of lower extremity eccentric muscle performance and loading. Thesis 1995. Karolinska Institutet. ISBN 91-628-1793-0.

36. Westblad P, Johansson C*. A reliable method for measuring eccentric and concentric knee extensor endurance. Eur J Exp Musculoskel Res 2: 151-157, 1993.

37. Westblad P, Tsai L, Johansson C*. Eccentric and concentric knee extensor performance in professional ballet dancers. Clin J Sports Med 5: 48-52, 1995.

38. Westblad P, Svedenhag J, Johansson C*. The validity of isokinetic knee extensor endurance measurements with reference to treadmill running capacities. Int J Sports Med 17 (2): 134-139, 1996.

39. Westing S, Seger J, Thorstensson A. Effects of electrical stimulation on eccentric and concentric torque velocity relationships during knee extension in man. Acta Physiol Scand 140: 17-22, 1990.

40. Winter D, Wells R, Orr G. Errors in the use of isokinetic dynamometers. Eur J Appl Physiol 46: 397-408, 1981.

41. Wredmark T, Törnqvist H, Johansson C*, Brobert B. Long-term results of the Bristow-Latarjet procedure for recurrent dislocation of the shoulder. Am J Sports Med 2: 157-161, 1992.

*"Johansson C" in the reference list is the same person as "Rolf C". The author changed "Johansson" to his family name "Rolf" in 1994. However, some of the papers published in 1995 are still under the former name.

G. Josef A. Salam

1. Introduction

In this section, I am going to evaluate the advantages of isokinetic technology, especially in the post-operative and post-traumatic stages. With careful and critical applications, isokinetics also plays a significant role in diagnosis and treatment.

The therapeutic application of isokinetic is controversial, and requires precise definition and great competence on the part of the therapist. Isokinetic movement patterns do not completely correspond to the natural movement patterns, therefore, need to be carefully and critically evaluated.

In rehabilitation, isokinetic methods are used as a supplement to physiotherapy, especially in CPM, and in concentric exercises. In athletic training, isokinetics is used in isolated movements to build a basis for subsequent training in specific sports.

Medical training therapy using isoinertial and isokinetic apparatus and exercise in therapeutic baths should improve: 1) muscular coordination, 2) strength, 3) endurance, 4) starting strength of single muscles, and 5) the function of all muscle chains involved in a particular movement.

2. Applications

The injured or operated joint is not exercised dynamically at first, but undergoes isometric training at various angles. Medical training therapy apparatus which can be fixed at any desired angle is used for this purpose (Figure 4-1).

When no cartilage damage has occurred to the tibial plateau, femoral condyles, or menisci, the entire extensor muscle chains can be trained within the range of motion allowed. Resistance is oriented to the release of pressure on the knee joint while walking. Conversely, when there has been no ligament damage, dynamic pressure load exercises in bending and extending the knee can be initiated, isokinetically at first, and then with freeweights.

As soon as possible, dynamic training procedures are started proximal and distal to the injured or operated joint, first isokinetically, and later isoinertially. Pure isoinertial training on the injured or operated limb, due to the nature of the resistance, can only be applied toward the end of the rehabilitation phase. Isokinetic therapy allows early dynamic pressure load, since the resistance applied to the greatest possible functional capacity of each muscle fiber involved at every angle. Contrary to isoinertial exercise training with weights, where resistance is fixed and speed is variable, in isokinetic exercise the opposite is true: speed is fixed, and resistance is variable (Table 4-5).

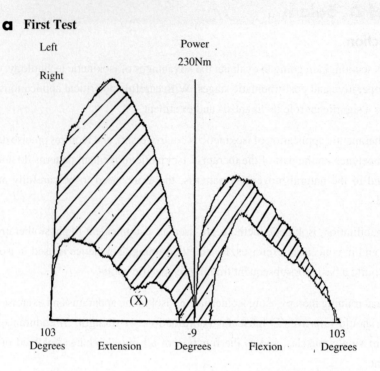

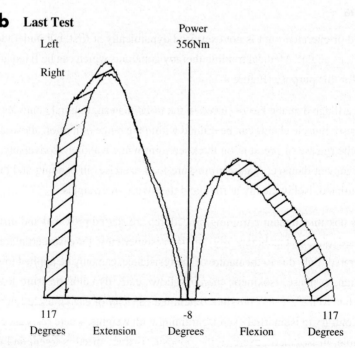

Figure 4-1 Isokinetic training after ACL reconstruction. a) first test: power deficit retropatellar pain (X); b) last test: deficit compensation.

Muscle Work	Speed	Resistance	Adjustment
Isometric	No	Variable	Fixed
Isoinertial	Variable	Constant	No
Isokinetic	Constant 0-500°/s	Variable	Absolute

Table 4-5 A comparison of the characteristics of three mode of muscle actions.

The speed at which the lever arm can be moved is fixed, ranging from 30°/s to 500°/s. Every increase in effort applied to the lever arm at any individual angular velocity setting proportionally increases the resistance (Figure 4-2).

Due to this variability in resistance, an affected joint cannot be overstrained, and the involved muscle fibers work maximally. Furthermore, variable resistance allows secure articular control during fast movements. This is not possible with weights. Using weights, uncontrollable and potentially injurious acceleration may take place. Furthermore, traditional weight training is limited by the weight and the weakest joint angle. The weaker muscle fibers quickly fatigued, since the resistance is not correspondingly reduced and an already damaged joint could be overloaded.

Acceleration forces may severely damage a joint during rehabilitation. These forces lie between 240Nm to 250Nm while walking, and raise to 1,500Nm to 3,000Nm while running. In top athletes, they can reach 6,000Nm. For this reason, a successful training program also has to take high acceleration forces into consideration, but in a controlled manner. This is only possible with the aid of isokinetics. For instance, when sprinting, a large number of muscle fibers must be recruited within 0.25 seconds from a complete standstill. Proper training attempts to: 1) overcome disturbances in the interaction between nervous and muscle systems controlling joint motions, and 2) create a fast and smooth muscular control system.

The faster this control system functions, the greater muscle potential can be developed from the moment of standstill. A muscle that has only been trained with isoinertial exercise does not contribute much, since it cannot reach its peak fast enough. Only a fast and smoothly-working muscle around the injured or operated joint can provide effective long-term protection to its ligaments and cartilage, thus exerting active arthritis prevention. The danger of re-injury can be avoided if ipsilateral muscle balance is maintained. Isokinetic diagnostics can uncover such weaknesses by the determination of peak torque acceleration energy. Isokinetic training, supported by certain coordination exercises in sprint training may alleviate such weaknesses. This therapy can be supported by neurophysiological techniques such as PNF and electrotherapy.

a

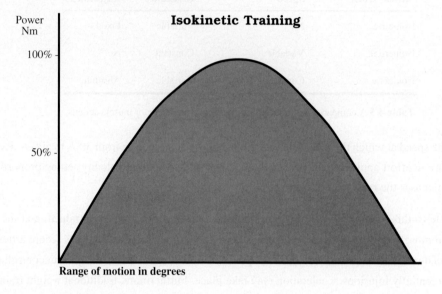

b

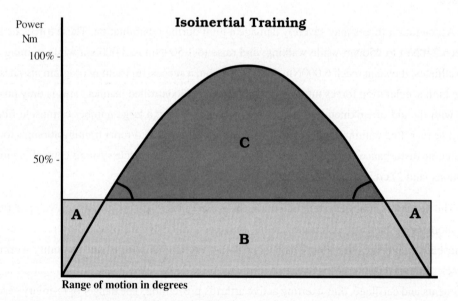

Figure 4-2 a) Isokinetic training: optimal power training, muscle functions 100%. b) Isoinertial training: (A) over-loaded joint and joint damage; (B) the stronger muscles are insufficiently trained; (C) the weaker muscles are quickly fatigued and not trained.

Improvements in operative techniques must be accompanied by improvements in rehabilitation techniques to give optimal results. For instance, reconstruction of the ACL was originally accomplished through arthrotomy. This required a period of rehabilitation ranging from 12 to 18 months. When isokinetic exercises were employed, rehabilitation was shortened to 6 to 9 months. With the present arthroscopically-assisted reconstruction, the procedure is even less invasive, and, again using isokinetic exercise, rehabilitation is shortened to 5 to 6 months.

In conclusion, being an orthopedic surgeon and the medical director of a modern rehabilitation center with isokinetic facilities, I believe that isokinetic techniques should be employed extensively for diagnosis and treatment of musculoskeletal injuries.

H. Kent E. Timm

Isokinetics continues to be controversial within the fields of Sports Medicine and orthopedic rehabilitation. The controversy is based upon the fundamental question of whether the relative advantages of isokinetic science and technology outweigh the relative disadvantages to establish a situation of clinical practicality for the treatment provider. Unfortunately, a definitive answer does not exist, and the decision on whether or not to utilize isokinetics is often left to the judgment of the individual clinician. However, a short review of the relative advantages and disadvantages of isokinetics may help to clarify the issue, and ensure that practitioners make an informed choice.

1. Advantages and disadvantages of isokinetics

The primary advantages of isokinetics lie in the areas of testing procedures and treatment effectiveness. Isokinetic testing is non-invasive and generates reliable data for the dynamic assessment of muscle performance of limbs and trunk. The accuracy of test data exceeds the results of isometric and isoinertial testing procedures. Isokinetic test methods have become a vital complement to the more traditional methods of physical examination, electromyography, and radiographic procedures in the assessment of patient with a neuromusculoskeletal disorder. As a treatment method, isokinetic exercise produces significant gains in strength, power, and endurance. These also have a positive carryover into increased concentric and eccentric functional muscle performance. Since isokinetics operates under the principle of accommodating resistance, such gains in muscle and functional performance are achieved through controlled loading of a joint system, which eliminates the risk of injury. Treatment programs which include isokinetics have demonstrated greater degree of short- and long-term clinical efficiency and cost effectiveness when compared to other methods of rehabilitation.

The major disadvantages of isokinetics are both economic and scientific. Isokinetic technology is still very expensive, and not all third-party reimbursement systems will pay for its use, which creates a fiscal detriment for its acquisition and use to clinicians. Also, functional practicality is an issue, as isokinetics still does not afford the diagnostic precision obtained through other methods of examination, such as MRI and arthroscopy. Also, it is clinically based, and it is not easily usable in a patient's environment of function, such as the football field or the basketball court. However, the primary problem is probably the lack of definitive knowledge on how to apply isokinetic science to the clinical context. The field still does not have a universal set of testing and rehabilitation procedures, even though isokinetics has been researched since 1967.

When considering isokinetics, it is hoped that the clinician will make a rational judgment on how and in what way to use isokinetics in his/her practice, rather than a simplistic "yes" or "no" decision. Isokinetics exists as a "tool" in each professional's "toolbox", which is the collection of different approaches and methods for the delivery of quality care to clients. Failure to weigh the relative liabilities against the potential advantages of isokinetics for patient's care, regardless of the actual outcome of the decision to use or not to use isokinetics, risks to compromise a clinician's professionalism and more importantly, the patient's treatment outcome.

2. Applications

In an attempt to find the balance between the relative advantages and disadvantages of isokinetics, a general paradigm has been developed for its application to patient care. The paradigm is designed to merge the aspects of isokinetic science and technology with the physiology of tissue response to injury or conditioning, to form a continuum with the general practice of orthopedic, rehabilitation and Sports Medicine. The continuum, shown in Table 4-6, does not require the use of isokinetics with each patient nor does it restrict the application of isokinetics to the listed areas: the individual needs of each patient always take precedence. This continuum has been effective for the successful treatment of a wide variety of patients with orthopedic and sports-related problems in the upper and lower extremities and in the lumbar spine.

Health status	Tissue status	Intervention	Isokinetics
Normal function	Normal function	Prevention	Testing
	Hypertrophy	Conditioning	Velocity spectrum
Injury	Inflammation	Medicine	Testing
		Surgery	
	Maturation	Rehabilitation	Short-arc exercise
	Remodelling	Rehabilitation	Velocity spectrum
Return to function	Remodelling	Rehabilitation	Velocity spectrum
	Normal function	Conditioning	Function specificity

Table 4-6 Continuum of care.

3. Future directions

The ongoing development of isokinetics will be determined by both economic and scientific influences. Regardless of the medical setting and of differences between various countries, market forces are demanding that the costs of health care decrease, while the quality of health care services is maintained, or increased. Isokinetics will continue to thrive in this environment if equipment manufacturers can produce leading edge technology that is, at the same time, affordable for the practitioner, and if the practitioner will continue to advance knowledge regarding the technology and its applications through clinical and laboratory research. Research is the actual key. Continued investigation should help to further refine the relatively recent advances in isokinetic knowledge: that shoulder rehabilitation does not require any isokinetic exercise other than internal and external rotation, and that lumbar spine testing beyond a single, patient-selected speed is unnecessary, and, thereby, further enhances the efficiency of treatment programs and the quality of functional outcomes for the patient. Such investigations will be facilitated through the newer designs of isokinetic systems, which have extensive research software for data collection built into the basic computer system. This allows comparisons of test results to normative databases via modem or the Internet, or direct correlation of isokinetic performance of exercising muscle groups to electromyographic activity or cardiovascular status. Work with these evolving forms of isokinetic technology should underscore the relative cost effectiveness of the intervention, thus helping to ensure the viability of isokinetics. However, regardless of cost or research, isokinetics should continue to be an important part of medical care as long as practitioners continue to address the specific needs of the individual patient and to regard isokinetics as a potential "tool" which could be selected from the professional "toolbox" for the management of orthopedic disorders and sports-related injuries.

Further Readings

1. Albert M. Eccentric Muscle Training in Sports and Orthopedics. 1991. NY : Churchill Livingstone, New York.

2. Davies GJ. A Compendium of Isokinetics in Clinical Usage and Rehabilitation Techniques. 4th edition, 1992. La Crosses, WI: S&S Publishers.

3. Davies GJ, Ellenbecker TS. Eccentric isokinetics. Orthop Phys Ther Clin North Am 1: 297-336, 1992.

4. Duncan PW, Chandler JM, Cavanaugh DK. Mode and speed specificity of eccentric and concentric exercise training. J Orthop Sports Phys Ther 11: 70-75, 1989.

5. Dvir Z. Isokinetics: Muscle Testing, Interpretation and Clinical Applications. 1995. NY: Churchill Livingstone, New York.

6. Ellenbecker TS, Davies GJ, Rowinski M. Concentric versus eccentric isokinetic strengthening of the rotator cuff: Objective data versus functional test. Am J Sports Med 16: 64-68, 1988.

7. Malone TR. Concentric isokinetics. Orthop Phys Ther Clin North Am 1: 283-296, 1992.

8. Perrin DH. Isokinetic Exercise and Assessment, 1993. Human Kinetics Publishers. Champaign, IL.

9. Timm KE. Clinical applications of a normative database for the Cybex TEF and TORSO spinal isokinetic dynamometers. Isokine Exerc Sci 5: 43-49, 1995.

10. Timm KE. Post-surgical knee rehabilitation: A 5-year study of four methods and 5,381 patients. Am J Sports Med 16: 463-468, 1988.

11. Timm KE. Investigation of the physiological overflow effect from speed-specific isokinetic activity. J Orthop Sports Phys Ther 9: 106-110, 1987.

12. Timm KE. Suggestion from the field: Isokinetic exercise to 50% fatigue. J Orthop Sports Phys Ther 8: 505-506, 1987.

13. Timm KE. Case study: Use of the Cybex II velocity spectrum in the rehabilitation of post-surgical knees. J Orthop Sports Phys Ther 6: 347-349, 1985.

14. Timm KE, Fyke D. The effect of test speed sequence on the concentric isokinetic performance of the knee extensor muscle group. Isokine Exerc Sci 3: 123-128, 1993

SECTION 3

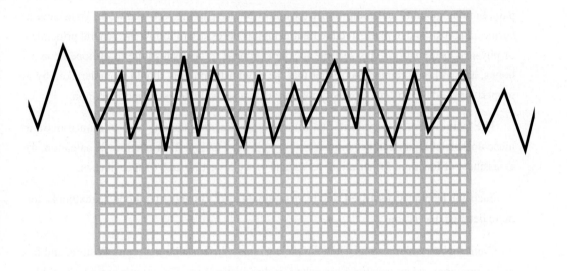

APPLICATIONS

V. Practical Applications of Isokinetics
A. Introduction

Few people undertake recreational or sports activities or any form of physical work without sustaining an acute or an overuse injury. Any structure of the musculoskeletal system may be involved. Many athletes who suffer from such injuries seek treatment from a Sports Medicine Physician, an Orthopedic Surgeon, a Physiotherapist, or an Athletic Trainer. Most of these ailments eventually heal with little or no medical care. However, some injuries cause significant pain, limiting mobility and compromise the ability to take part in sports and work. To achieve a correct diagnosis and to plan effective treatment, it is necessary to follow the general principles of physical examination. This section does not propose to be a substitute to orthopedic textbooks, and will only remind the reader that the diagnostic process should be undertaken by a properly trained health care provider, possibly with a special interest in sports trauma.

The principles of physical examination in the assessment and evaluation of a musculoskeletal injury can be summarized in 1) history taking, 2) inspection, 3) palpation, 4) assessment of function, 5) sensation, reflex and vascular testing, and 6) special tests.

Each will be briefly discussed, and readers should refer to standard orthopedic textbooks for more detailed discussion.

Clinical observation begins when the patient enters the consultation room. Posture, and facial expressions, when questions are asked or diagnostic maneuver are performed, should be noted. The presence of compensatory movements, and the ability to change position comfortably are all important parts of physical examination.

1. History taking

The art of history taking should be patiently developed as students, first, and as practitioners, for the rest of one's life. A history well taken will give the diagnosis away, and the rest of the physical examination will be performed to confirm any suspicions. However, one should keep an open mind. Although a twisting injury of the knee in a football player may result in haemarthrosis, which is indicative of a torn anterior cruciate ligament in 70% of cases, it should be remembered that a peripheral detached meniscus can cause the same picture, and carry a totally different prognosis.

At least part of the clinical history can be obtained before actually seeing the patient if structured questionnaires are used. In Sports Medicine, the practitioner should be aware of the structure of the game, and, in team sports, of the specific requirements of each playing position. Equipment, playing surface and handedness should be noted, together with the level of training and competition. Previous injuries, any medications taken and the use of performance enhancing drugs should be investigated. The time of the day and the dietary practices can give clues to the underlying causes, and illness can account for undue tiredness or carelessness. The athlete should be asked to describe the mechanism of injury, and the sensations following the injury. Not all serious injuries are immediately disabling. For example, an athlete with an acutely torn anterior cruciate ligament can return to play immediately, only to find later that a painful haemarthrosis has developed. The age of the athlete plays a role. In children, anterior cruciate ligament injuries are uncommon, and, if they occur, they more frequently involve the bone-ligament junction, instead of being mid-substance as in adults.

It is always worthwhile asking the patient whether diagnostic tests have been performed elsewhere, thus avoiding duplications. Finally, the attitude of the patient toward the injury should be noted.

2. Inspection

The first and paramount rule is to achieve adequate exposure. Comparison with the uninjured side should be performed, and differences in shape and contour should be noted. The presence of swelling and redness is often indices of inflammation, and scars may be due to previous injuries treated operatively. Discolorations may give away the use of cortico-steroid injections for treatment. Information of observed surface anatomy irregularities, such as asymmetry and atrophy, should be recorded. Posture should be compared with normal posture. Bony and soft tissues landmarks should be appreciated and compared.

3. Palpation

Palpation should be undertaken with gentle but firm hand, keeping in mind that the aim is not to inflict pain, but to ascertain facts. Following a planned sequence, palpation should assess the individual joints, the various muscles, and the course and insertion of the tendons. Also, the areas of discomfort should be identified. During palpation, the examiner should note changes in temperature. An increase may indicate inflammation, a decrease vascular impairment. It should be remembered that, physiologically, the local temperature over a joint is a few degrees lower than the surrounding muscles. As each joint is examined, symmetry, congruity, discomfort, laxity, and audible and palpable crepitating should be noted.

The full length of the muscle, including the musculo-tendinous junction, should be palpated, possibly both in the resting and in a stretched position. Atrophy should be noted, and a cause sought.

4. Assessment of function

Active and passive motion should be examined, and, if possible, individual muscles should be examined. The range of motion, both active and passive, possible discomfort associated with motion, the ability to move against resistance, and the strength developed should be recorded. At this point, isokinetic techniques assist in quantifying muscle strength. For clinical muscle testing, the examiner may choose to apply resistance in one of three ways: 1) during an isometric contraction at a given angle, 2) throughout the whole range of motion, or 3) in a break-type test. Also, placement of the resistance can be varied. Toward the end of the examination, some functional tests can be administered, if pain allows. Concentric and eccentric control should be observed.

When completed, functional data coupled with history, inspection and palpation should give a fairly precise picture of the patient's problem, and form the basis for a critical assessment of the athlete's presenting problem.

5. Sensation, vascular and reflex testing

Comments on changes in sensation should be noted. A systematic bilateral assessment of the dermatomes of the involved area should be performed using a sharp and a blunt instrument. Coupling the findings of sensation testing with muscle testing may help in directing or confirming a clinical suspicion. Palpation of peripheral pulses should be routinely undertaken. Reflex testing of the relevant muscles should be undertaken, possibly extending the examination to a full neurological and vascular examination.

6. Special tests

After the completion of the clinical evaluation, the need for further tests is determined. These may include various forms of imaging, electrophysiological tests, arteriography, and Doppler ultrasonography. Functional performance can be assessed by video tapes of the injured athlete, and the tapes can be used to assess the impact of treatment on the athlete.

In this area, isokinetic testing should be considered to assess and quantify muscular performance. Some pathologies may affect muscle strength in a particular range, and hence specific training is required; otherwise recurrence is highly likely.

B. Variables commonly measured with isokinetic dynamometry

In the following paragraphs, a definition of each of the variables commonly measured in isokinetic testing will be given, with a comment on its usefulness and validity.

1. Torque

Torque is the turning effect (or moment) of a force on an object (torque [Nm or ft-lb] = force [N] x distance from axis of rotation [m]). In isokinetic dynamometry, the axis of rotation is the axis of the dynamometer.

a. Peak torque

Peak torque (PT, unit: Nm) is the most commonly measured strength variable in isokinetic testing. It is the single highest torque output produced by muscle contraction as the limb moves through the ROM (Figure 5-1). Its measurement is both accurate and reproducible, and, being the most frequently used variable, it is often considered the gold standard in isokinetic evaluation (Kannus 1994). Clinically, it is important because bilateral torque curves and ipsilateral agonist/antagonist torque curves are compared to assess muscle symmetry and/or the success of a given rehabilitation program.

b. Mean peak torque

PT describes the muscle's force-generating capacity. Mean peak torque (MPT, unit: Nm) is the average torque over a given number of repetitions. This is a good test of the overall function of the muscle, because function is dependent on the subject's ability to repeat movements (Urquhart et al 1995). The effects of fatigue may, however, confuse the results. When measuring PT, five contractions are commonly taken to ensure reliability. It is not uncommon to ignore the first contraction because it sometimes deviates excessively from the other measurements. For this reason, MPT is sometimes seen as a less meaningful variable. It is therefore auspicable that all repetitions are maximal.

c. Peak torque to weight ratio

To compare test results between individuals, PT can be expressed by per kilogram body mass, commonly termed as peak torque to weight ratio (PTW). Muscle strength is largely dependent on its cross-sectional area (Astrand and Rodahl 1986). On average, men have a larger

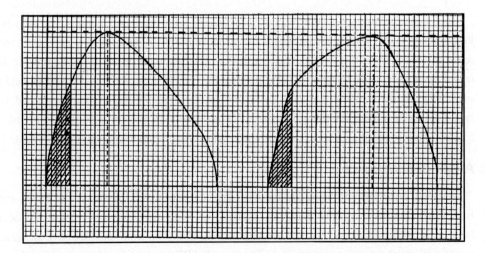

Figure 5-1 Peak Torque (PT) at two different angles. In the diagram on the left, PT occurs at an earlier angle than in the diagram on the right.

muscle mass as well as a greater peak torque to weight ratio. Only lower body measurements are expressed in relation to body weight, as the lower limbs are weight-bearing. Athletes and players engaged in explosive sports require a high PT and therefore a higher PTW ratio which will enable fast acceleration of the body mass. Endurance athletes require a relatively low PT, and thus a lower PTW.

d. Angle-specific torque

Angle-specific torque (AST, unit: Nm) describes the torque generated at specific angles, other than the peak. It may be used to evaluate the optimum joint angle for maximum force production. This is important when comparing the strength of agonist and antagonist muscle groups at a particular angle of joint motion. Unfortunately, the reliability of AST has been shown to be good only when torque is measured from relatively central locations in the ROM. AST reliability decreases dramatically when measured more peripherally (Kannus and Kaplan 1991).

2. Time to peak torque

Time to peak torque (unit: seconds) describes the ability to produce torque rapidly. It is of interest when assessing athletes who require explosive power. If time to peak torque is prolonged, it may indicate that the recruitment of type II (fast) fibers is suboptimal (Kannus 1994). Time to peak torque is not of such great interest if peak torque acceleration energy can be measured. The latter may be more useful in the assessment of athletes engaged in explosive sports.

3. Torque-velocity ratio

In concentric isokinetic exercise, torque decreases with increasing angular velocity. Peak torque tends to stay almost unchanged between the angular velocities of 0°/s and 60°/s, and it tends to decline thereafter with increased velocity. The decline is due to changing muscle fiber recruitment patterns. Both type I and II fibers are maximally activated at lower speeds, and the increasing angular velocity results in smaller and smaller fiber populations being recruited, with type I fibers becoming relatively inactive (Kannus 1994). In eccentric exercise, instead, the torque remains the same or increases with increasing velocity up to a point (Perrin 1993).

4. Angle of occurrence

Angle of occurrence refers to the angle (in degrees) at which PT occurs in the ROM, and it is routinely reported in isokinetic studies (Figure 5-2). With increasing test velocity, PT occurs later in the ROM. It seems that, at high angular velocities, the limb may not have an optimal joint position for muscular performance. The recorded PT may not therefore represent the subject's maximum torque-producing capacity (Osternig 1986). Also, the weaker the muscle, the later PT tends to occur, possibly because of slow neural recruitment (Kannus and Järvinen

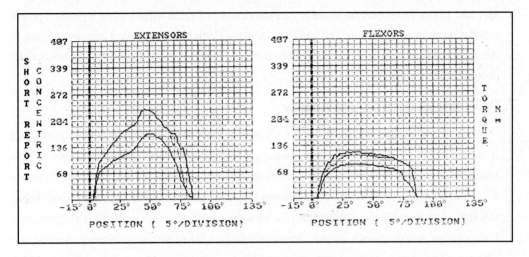

Figure 5-2 The angle at which the single highest point occurs is the angle of occurrence.

1990). The reliability of the angle of occurrence is often unacceptably low (Kannus 1994) because of the difficulty in achieving standard joint alignment in repeated testing.

5. Total work

In isokinetics, work is defined as the area under the torque versus angular displacement (time) curve. Work (unit: joules J) is torque multiplied by angular distance, and total work (TW) is the sum of all the work performed in all the pre-selected test repetitions (Hislop and Perrine 1967). It is considered by some as a measure of endurance of the muscle group tested. It may be difficult to differentiate between genuine muscle weakness and lack of endurance from this measure. Nevertheless, with improved muscle strength and/or endurance, the total work done will also increase.

Peak work (PW), on the other hand, is the work done during the best test repetition, and it is sometimes referred to best work repetition (BWR). Both TW and PW have been shown to be consistent and reliable. Because both can be calculated from PT, their clinical usefulness has been questioned (Kannus 1994).

6. Peak power and average power

Peak power (PP, unit: Watts = joules/second) output is the highest power output achieved during the best repetition divided by the movement time. Whereas torque declines, power production rises as angular velocity increases during isokinetic exercise (Osternig 1986). Average power (AP, unit: W and J/s) refers to the total work performed during the given contractions, divided by the actual total movement time. The use of PP and AP in routine testing is not common mainly because these can easily be calculated from PT (Kannus 1990, Kannus and

Järvinen 1989). As an exception, these measures can be of value when testing high level power athletes, such as weightlifters and sprinters. Kannus (1994) recommended that, in addition to AP measurement with athletes, the whole power-velocity curve with a range of test speeds should be determined.

7. Peak torque acceleration energy

Peak torque acceleration energy (PKTAE, unit: J) is the greatest amount of work performed in the first 125ms (1/8 sec) of a single torque production in the test repetition. It gives an estimate of the speed or rate of torque production and therefore reflects "explosive power" (Figure 5-3). Such measurement would be of interest in testing athletes involved in explosive events. Recently, however, Kannus (1994) has criticized the use of this measure for two main reasons. First, at slow speeds, results showed unacceptable variability and inconsistency. Second, the whole concept of "torque acceleration energy" has been questioned because it appears to lack a basis from Newtonian physics (Perrin et al 1989, Rothstein et al 1987). In general evaluation, however, the higher the PKTAE, the greater the explosive power tends to be.

8. Endurance ratios/indices

Isokinetic muscle endurance is generally measured in three different ways: 1) the number of repetitions of maximum effort test movements required to produce a 50% drop in torque output; 2) the percent declined in work, torque or power output from the beginning to the end of a predetermined time period, such as 30s or 45s, or after a set number of repetitions, for example, fifty contractions; and 3) comparison of work done during the first five and last five repetitions. Figure 5-4 shows a measure of muscle endurance.

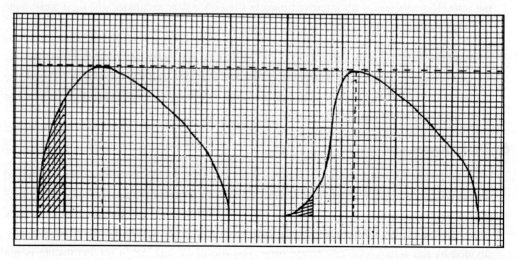

Figure 5-3 The shaded areas under the curves denote the first 125 ms of a single torque production and the PKTAE.

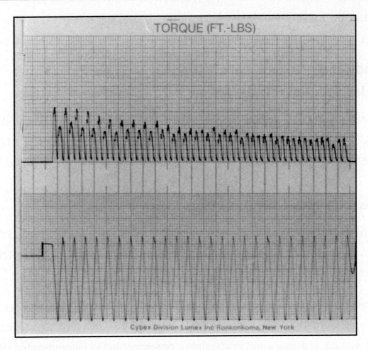

Figure 5-4 An example of an endurance ratio curve.

Absolute endurance measures (eg, work in a 25-repetition test) appear to be consistent enough for clinical and scientific use, and for documenting progress in endurance training (Kannus 1994). On the other hand, relative endurance measures (eg, work during the last five repetitions divided by work during the first five repetitions) are relatively less sensitive to changes in training status, and show a less test-re-test reproducibility (Kannus 1994). However, relative endurance is still the most commonly used and a popular way of measuring endurance, possibly due to similar problems which occur with the other ways of measuring endurance.

C. Practical procedures in isokinetic measurement

The reliability and validity of isokinetic measurements, like any other measurements in clinical practice and especially in research, are dependent on carefully standardized pre-test procedures. This ensures that intraindividual and interindividual test-re-test results can be compared and/or pooled together. In the following paragraphs, we will describe contraindications to isokinetic testing, and detail general pre-test procedures.

1. Indications to isokinetic testing

Isokinetic testing is employed to assist in the detection of strengths and weaknesses in the musculature around a given joint. It is also used to establish baseline values to help in the assessment of the extent of an injury, and for the subsequent construction of a rehabilitation program.

2. Contraindications to isokinetic testing

a. Relative contraindications

The tested joint must be examined thoroughly for habitual subluxation and dislocation before testing. If the patient suffers from acute muscle spasms and has restricted ROM because of inflammation (eg, rheumatoid arthritis) or acute effusion (eg, sprained ankle), the test should be postponed.

b. Absolute contraindications

In conditions such as joint instability, fractures, severe osteoporosis around the joint to be tested, acute swelling, bone or joint malignancy, or immediately after surgical procedures, such as ACL reconstruction, isokinetic testing must not be employed (Table 5-1).

Pre-screening health questionnaire should reveal information on any existing cardiovascular (CV) problems. For individuals who appear to be at risk of such problems (aged over 40 men or aged 50 women, sedentary and overweight), pre-screening is recommended (Rantanen et al 1995, Richter 1992, Eckhardt et al 1991). Richter (1992) recommended that patients receiving anticoagulant therapy for cerebral, cardiac, or venous conditions may be at risk for complications.

Relative contraindications	Absolute contraindications
Pain	Soft tissue healing constraints
Limited ROM	Severe pain
Effusion or synovitis	Extremely limited ROM
Chronic third degree sprain	Severe effusion
Subacute strain (musculo-tendinous unit)	Fractures
	Acute strain (musculo-tendinous unit)
	Acute sprain

Table 5-1 Relative and absolute contraindications to isokinetic testing (Adapted from Davies. A Compendium of Isokinetics in Clinical Usage and Rehabilitation Techniques, 2nd edition, 24, 1984).

3. Timing of the test

There are no standard guidelines for starting isokinetic conditioning after an injury or surgery. Much depends on the type of injury, degree of damage and the extent of the surgery. The clinician has to strike a balance between two factors. On one hand, overexerting a tissue which has not healed may hinder the healing process, and even set it back. On the other hand, imposing stress on the healing tissue in an optimal and progressive manner will aid healing. Generally, the timing of isokinetic testing and training must consider the nature and anatomical location of the injury or dysfunction, and the therapeutic procedure (surgical/non-surgical) followed (Urquhart et al 1995, Sherman et al 1982). As a general guideline, patients able to perform a grade 3 movement (MRC grading, from zero to 5), ie, movement against gravity, can be tested. In such cases, testing must involve high speeds (180°/s). Where grade 2+ movement is possible, isokinetics should be restricted to CPM only. Gravity eliminated exercises would only be indicated. These guidelines are conservative, yet safe.

4. Practicalities of isokinetic testing
a. Pre-test procedures
(1) Patient information

Explain what is required from the subject (Figure 5-5). Explain what isokinetic concentric and eccentric actions mean and how they may possibly feel during a test. Advise the patient that the dynamometer is set at a certain velocity and that the resistance will vary according to the force applied by it. Describe and demonstrate that the machine will push or pull their limbs,

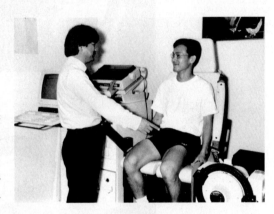

Figure 5-5 Explaining isokinetic concentric and eccentric actions to the subject before the test.

and that they should resist this as hard as possible. Also, clarify the possible after-effects of isokinetic exercise, especially the likelihood of DOMS.

(2) Familiarization

Let the subject "play" with the machine first using submaximal and then maximal force, at different speeds. Familiarization, especially with eccentric actions, may be time consuming, but essential to obtain reliable and reproducible results. Should the individual subject require it, the first session should be spent on practising and the test be done in the second session. We recommend a separate familiarization session, particularly when research work is planned. Generally, prior to actual testing, three submaximal and three maximal repetitions have been found adequate for obtaining reliable measurements of isokinetic PT, work and power (Perrin 1986).

(3) General warm-up and stretching

A 10- to 15-minute warm-up, including rhythmic submaximal exercise, such as rope skipping, running on the spot or cycle ergometry, is followed by a standardized set of static stretching of the muscles around the joints to be tested.

(4) Body positioning and joint alignment

It is essential to locate the best possible axis of rotation for each joint to allow maximum

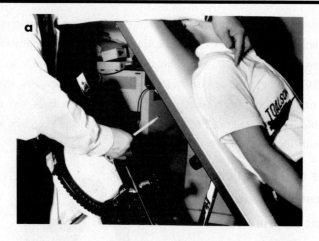

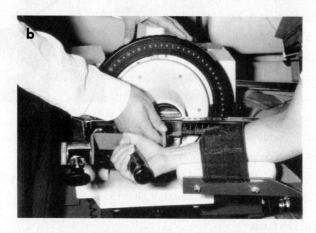

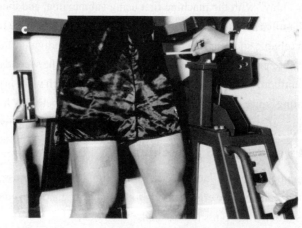

Figure 5-6 Aligning the joint movement axes and the axis of the dynamometer according to the joint and the motion plane to be tested. a) positioning of the shoulder joint for abduction/adduction; b) the joint axis of the wrist; c) the trunk flexion/extension test.

functional ROM. This can be done by palpating the anatomical landmarks around the joint. Careful alignment will ensure smooth, comfortable and safe motion for the subject. It is essential that the muscles being tested are in a semi-relaxed position to enable a maximal contraction of the given muscles. During upper body testing, other than shoulder internal/external rotation in modified neutral position, which is done from a standing position, the feet should be in a non-weight bearing position. The unaffected limb or, in normal subjects, the dominant limb is tested first. This will aid familiarization with the movement pattern, the test requirements, and help in accommodating the resistance without apprehension (Figure 5-6).

(5) Stabilization

This will ensure that the muscle group to be tested is well isolated, and that the contribution from accessory muscles will be minimal. It is also easier to avoid trick movements. Stabilization occurs both at the waist and the chest, in addition to the joint area to be tested (Figure 5-7). If the lower limbs are tested, the arms will be crossed and kept across the chest or, as in some dynamometers, firmly hold the handles provided. Gripping the sides is recommended when measuring the quadriceps femoris isokinetic torque (Hinton 1988) and is likely to

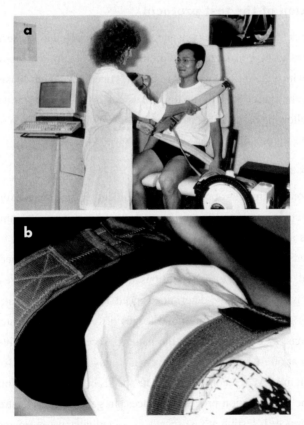

Figure 5-7 a) Strapping for stability prior to a knee test. b) Strapping the trunk for stability prior to all upper limb tests.

improve subsquent PT measurement. During upper limb testing, the feet should be in a non-weight-bearing position. It is important to realize that insufficient padding or too tightly fitted belts may cause discomfort, and thus inhibit force production. The belt should be felt firm but comfortable throughout the whole test. Communication with the subject is essential.

(6) Gravity correction

Gravity correction is applied when assessing the limb through a gravity-dependent position, such as knee flexion/extension. This will account for the weight of the dynamometer's lever arm and the limb being tested. Acceleration of the limb due to gravity will artificially inflate subsequent torque output and vice versa. This is particularly important when assessing reciprocal muscle group ratios, such as the hamstring/quadriceps ratio (Kannus 1994, Westing and Seger 1989, Figoni et al 1988), or the shoulder abduction/adduction and hip flexion/extension. Gravity correction is not required for ankle dorsiflexion/plantarflexion, shoulder internal/external rotation and trunk flexion/extension.

b. The test protocol

(1) Selection of the test protocol

This will be determined by the type and severity of injury, and the surgical procedure used. The main factors to be considered include the mode, velocity and duration of contractions, ROM through which the muscle work is to be performed, the length-tension relationship of the muscle group to be exercised, and flexion and extension cycles with or without pause between cycles. In the following paragraphs, we provide some practical advice on what to consider when deciding upon test protocols.

(a) Velocity and duration

The conditioning stimulus appears to be dependent on time spent exercising rather than on the number of repetitions, and 30 seconds are required to induce a training effect (Costill et al 1979). Exercise at slow speeds through a given ROM will take longer time to complete than exercise at faster speeds. As a general guideline, repetitions are determined in relation to the test speed employed: at 60°/s, five to six repetitions and at 180°/s, twenty-five repetitions per set are required. Force is applied at a pre-determined speed, keeping in mind that, at slower speeds, the force exerted is greater. During the initial stages of rehabilitation, faster speeds are used in concentric actions, as this is safer for the patient. Eccentric movements are done at slower speeds, starting at 60°/s, as fast speed movements may be dangerous; for example, they may damage the graft in an ACL reconstruction. The speeds in concentric training are then gradually decreased as the rehabilitation process advances. In general, muscle strength testing at slow speeds always proceeds testing at fast speeds as it facilitates warm-up and aids in the learning process, particularly in inexperienced subjects.

(b) ROM and length-tension relationship

Unless an injury prevents it, a muscle should be trained and tested through its whole available range, reflecting the patient's daily or sporting activities. It is also worth noting that hyperextension will decrease subsequent power output as dictated by the length-tension relationship. Trick movements will also be encouraged by hyperextension.

(c) Agonist/antagonist cycle

In general, when testing concentric flexion/extension, a pause is built in because the antagonist relaxes while the agonist contracts. Therefore, no pause will be required. When testing concentric/eccentric actions of the same muscle group, a small pause (about one second) is recommended.

(d) Order of tests

Strength and power tests are normally done before endurance tests to avoid undue fatigue.

(2) Actual test protocol

(a) Warm-up

Each test testing session will begin with a warm-up including submaximal and maximal repetitions. Each test speed should be preceeded by a warm-up of at least three repetitions. In our laboratory, we use seven to ten repetitions and more, if needed. This helps the patient to familiarize with the speeds to be employed. While the patient will get used to the machine set-up, this also helps to ensure comfortable and unrestricting positioning.

(b) Test velocity

The test velocities normally used for the different body parts are presented in Section 1, Table 2-2 .

(c) Number of test repetitions

Peak torque: Two to six contractions at a given velocity are generally recommended. Five are normally used in our laboratory.

Endurance: Twenty-five contractions at the given velocity.

(d) Rest

A predetermined rest interval follows each test repetition and each set of repetitions. After five maximal repetitions, 30- to 60-second rest is sufficient, while more than 60 seconds may be required after an endurance test of twenty-five repetitions. A one-minute rest is taken between different speeds. Three to 5 minutes are allowed between testing of opposite sides. Preferably, no two lower/upper limb tests, ie, knee and ankle, should be performed on the same day to avoid undue fatigue. If this is impractical, an hour's rest before the next test is necessary.

(3) Special considerations

(a) Verbal encouragement

Verbal encouragement has been shown to affect test results, and thus must be standardized both in research and in test-re-test situations, if at all used. Some authors use verbal encouragement throughout the test, while others instruct the patient to produce maximum effort before each set of test repetitions.

(b) Visual feedback

Visual feedback of both slow and fast isokinetic testing influences subsequent test results, increasing the torque output. Timm (1988) has suggested that letting patients see the torque curve may be distracting and should be avoided. Any visual feedback should be standardized.

(c) Time of day

The time of testing should be kept within 30 minutes of the same time of the day to ensure that results are comparable (Wyse et al 1994). For maximal leg strength values, the measurement should be made close to 18:00 to 19:30 hours as this appears to be the optimal time for producing maximal force.

(d) Testing frequency

Frequency of testing depends on the muscle group being trained. In rehabilitation, once per month is sufficient, whereas athletic monitoring may be less frequent.

D. Common problems with testing

1. Problems related to the patient

1) Isokinetic movements are "unnatural" and require some practice, although they may be perceived as easy (Figure 5-8). It is important to deliver clear instructions and to make sure that the patient understands them, especially when testing eccentric movements;

2) Subjects think that they have exerted maximum effort when they clearly have not;

3) Unfit subjects may feel physically sick after a test; and

4) Subjects often sweat considerably during a test which makes them feel uncomfortable during the second half of the test.

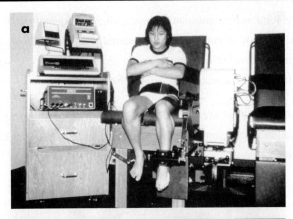

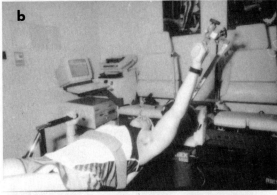

Figure 5-8 a) The knee extension is an unfamiliar movement for a gymnast. b) Testing for the shoulder extension. A basketball player never throws a ball in lying position with the back supported.

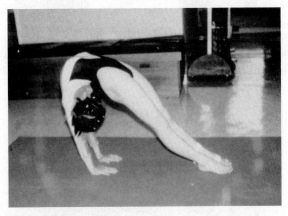

Figure 5-9 A young Asian gymnast.

2. Problems related to the machine

1) The dimensions of the machine make isokinetic testing and exercise unsuitable for many Asian subjects and for young children (Figure 5-9);

2) Some of the joint movements cannot be stabilized adequately with some of the available dynamometers. For instance, internal/external rotation of the shoulder in neutral position, and ankle dorsiflexion/plantarflexion tend to be difficult. Stabilization will affect the reliability of the measurement (Figure 5-10);

3) Some of the joint axes are difficult to align in a repeatable way, such as in shoulder abduction/adduction testing (Figure 5-11). When testing the ankle, an oblique axis is required; and

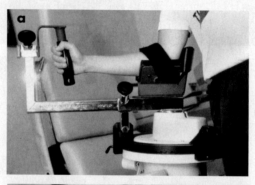

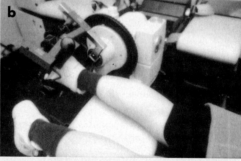

Figure 5-10 a) The shoulder internal/external rotation test at neutral shoulder position has little strapping to provide stabilization. b) The ankle dorsiflexion/plantarflexion test has no fixation to the ankle. Straps are placed around the thigh.

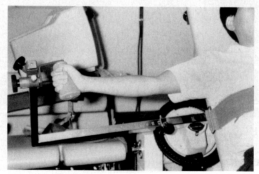

Figure 5-11 Aligning for shoulder abduction/adduction testing. The dynamometer has to be tilted at an angle parallel to the shaft of the applicator.

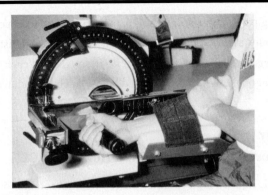

Figure 5-12 The ROM of the wrist joint is physiologically limited.

4) Large or small joints, such as the hip and the wrist, tend to give less reliable measurements (Perrin 1993) (Figure 5-12). Advances in stabilization techniques have recently been introduced by the manufacturers of the Kin-Com.

3. Problems related to the operator

1) The operator needs to be experienced with the testing procedures to provide an efficient, reliable and effective service; and

2) Sometimes the patient's performance fluctuates greatly and it may be difficult to determine when to stop and repeat a test.

E. Interpretation of isokinetic curve data

When investigating a pathological condition, the test curve is compared to that produced by the unaffected side, or to population norms, should the condition be present in both limbs. We would like to emphasize again that torque curves can only be used as a supplementary aid in formulating a diagnosis of a condition.

Following the test, inspect the data or torque curves for the following:

1) Reliability of the PT, to see if most of the repetitions produce similar curves;

2) Any markedly outlying data, for example, bilateral discrepancy of 200% or endurance ratio of over 100%; and

3) The torque curve for normal or expected appearance.

In the following paragraphs, normal and pathological torque curves will be presented for a number of commonly assessed conditions. Torque curve characteristics and pathomechanics leading to variations in the torque curve will be described for each of the conditions. More detailed information on the conditions outlined below can be found, for example, in DeLee and Drez (1994).

1. Knee pathology

a. Anterior cruciate ligament insufficiency (ACLI)

Definition: ACL injuries are caused by forced internal rotation of the tibia relative to the femur due to forceful twisting, impact to one side of the knee, or impact causing hyperextension or hyperflexion. ACL injuries are common in contact sports and Alpine skiing (Peterson and Renström 1986).

Characteristics: There is a plateau or a double peak with deformation that occurs in the mid portion of the knee extension. Figure 2-6 in Section 1 shows a sample diagram of an unaffected quadriceps/hamstrings torque and Figure 5-13 shows the torque curve of an ACLI knee.

Pathomechanics: The ACL provides the helicoid guiding action of the knee through the ROM and the anterior and anterior lateral rotational instability (ALRI) translations which occur in mid-range (Figure 5-13). Injury to the ligament produces a mechanical dysfunction which results in the deformation seen in the torque curve.

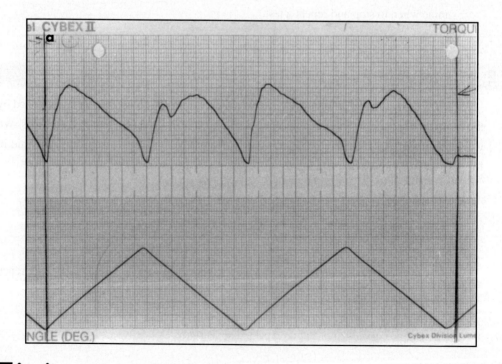

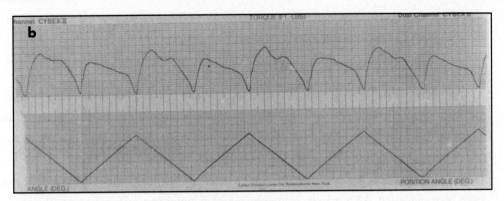

Figure 5-13 a) and b) CDRC curves of a knee with ACLI.

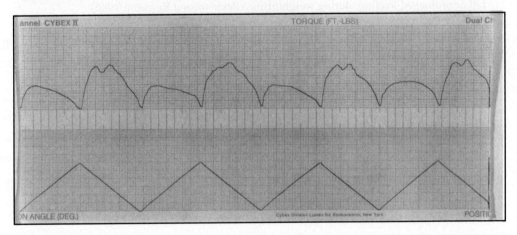

Figure 5-14 A curve demonstrating a meniscus injury.

b. Meniscus lesions

Definition: The menisci consist of a semilunar fibrocartilage, partly filling the space between the femoral and tibial articular surfaces. Their function is to stabilize the joint. They serve as shock absorbers between the tibia and the femur. Meniscus lesions are common in contact sports and they often occur in combination with ligamentous injuries. They are caused by twisting impact to the knee and hyperextension and flexion. Varying degrees of rupture occurs through the meniscal tissue (Peterson and Renström 1986).

Characteristics: The time rate of tension development (TRTD) is normal in this condition. A double hump on the curve including a W-shaped wave within this hump is evident (Figure 5-14).

Pathomechanics: Some patients with meniscus lesions will demonstrate the above abnormality caused by compression or pinching of the torn meniscus. The wave pattern may be associated with abnormal areas of compression or reflex inhibition. Generally, the PT appears lower on the affected than on the unaffected side. It should be remembered that a normal isokinetic test result does not exclude meniscal pathology.

c. Anterior knee pain (AKP)

Definition: An umbrella definition, it most often involves unspecified damages to the articular surface of the patella which causes pains, particularly when walking down the stairs and squatting. Compared with the normal flexion of the joint on flat ground, knee flexion increases considerably during, for example, normal walking, increasing the compression forces between patella and femur. The exact etiology of AKP is often unclear, and many contributing factors have been suggested. AKP may be caused by repeated minor or a major impact to the knee, a fall or prolonged loading, during weightlifting (Peterson and Renstöm 1986).

Characteristics: Extension torque is significantly decreased with a plateau occurring through the mid-ROM. A wavy pattern characterizes the plateau as seen in Figure 5-15. The flexion curve may be normal.

Pathomechanics: The main reason behind the shape of the extension curve is pain inhibition. Because of underlying pathology, greater amount of stress is transmitted to the innervated subchondral bone, causing pain. The shape of the torque curve may also be a consequence of articular cartilage damage and irregularity on the joint surface. Such anterior knee pain normally does not affect performance in flexion.

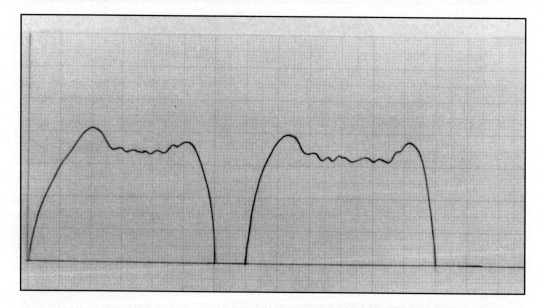

Figure 5-15 An isokinetic curve produced by a patient with chondromalacia patella.

d. Patella subluxation

Definition: Dislocation of the patella usually occurs laterally, often as a result of violent impact. Fragments of bone and cartilage may be dislodged and become loose in the joint, and a tear of the joint capsule medial to the patella may occur. Patella subluxation causes impaired mobility, bleeding and tenderness (Peterson and Renström 1986).

Characteristics: Figure 5-16 shows a double-humped curve, where the first hump is always higher. These humps are relatively further apart if compared to the double peaked seen with ACL insufficiency.

Pathomechanics: At the start of the test, the knee is flexed to 90° and the patella firmly seated in the femoral sulcus. When the knee is extended, at around 30° of flexion, subluxation will normally occur, resulting in an irregular torque curve.

Figure 5-16a: At the point where the patella subluxes, pain causes momentary inhibition, reflected in the downward drop of the curve. As extension continues, the patella relocates, and additional torque is produced, as shown in the slight upward turn in the curve. The humps tend to be relatively far apart, reflecting the time that the patient takes to redevelop the level of force exerted initially.

Figure 5-16b: Similar to Figure 5-16a, where the patella subluxation causes mechanical dysfunction in the extensor mechanism, reducing the force generating capacity of the quadricep. Pain may also be partially responsible.

Figure 5-16c: The sharp peak seen in the torque curve signifies general weakness in the whole of the quadriceps group, especially in the vastus medialis, causing a rapid drop in force production, particularly toward the end of ROM. The curve is unable to maintain its normally rounded shape, which is reflected in a weak PT and a poor work output.

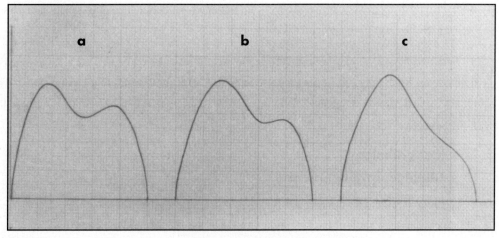

Figure 5-16 a) to c)Typical curves produced by a patient with patella subluxation.

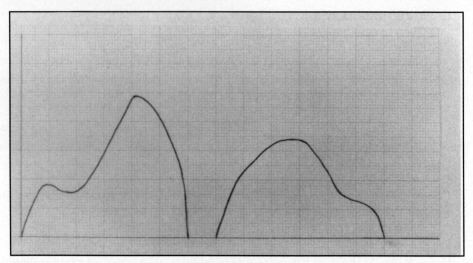

Figure 5-17 Isokinetic curve from a pateint's knee affected by osteochondritis dissecans.

e. Osteochondritis dissecans

Definition: Often defined as a stress fracture at the joint surface, it commonly affects the knee. The underlying causes are not well defined, and a discrete piece of articular cartilage and its subchondral bone may become detached from the surrounding cartilage. When this happens, a loose body is released into the joint involved, causing damage to the articular cartilage. The loose body may cause locking of the joint, and recurrent effusion. These episodes are often accompanied by significant pain (Peterson and Renström 1986). The curves described here refer to osteochondritis dissecans in the knee.

Characteristics: As seen in Figure 5-17, the early part the torque curve of the quadriceps shows deformation and flattening. A similar deformation can be seen in the hamstrings curve. Both the hamstrings and quadriceps curves are flattened, reflecting pain. Deformation occurs in both curves because of the articular involvement.

Pathomechanics: Abnormal pressure in the area of articulation causes the changes seen in both curves. Sometimes, these are angle-specific and affect both limbs to the same extent. The torque curve deviation is repeated, and, for example, the Cybex II+ shows a mirror image in the torque curve.

2. Shoulder pathology

a. Shoulder impingement

Definition: Shoulder impingement is caused by trapping of the rotator cuff between the head of humerus and the vault of the acromion process of the scapula and the coraco-acromial ligament. Any inflammation, calcification and thickening of ligaments or tendons will cause irritation and painful inflammation. Shoulder impingement is common in tennis players, swimmers, throwers and weightlifters who perform repetitive movements of the arms in or above the horizontal plane (Peterson and Renström 1986).

Characteristics: With shoulder impingement syndromes, a sharp and significant drop can be seen in the mid-range of abduction/adduction (Figure 5-18a). In flexion, a drop appears at the initial range (Figure 5-18b), and at 90° external/internal rotation, the PT will not necessarily be low (Figure 5-18c).

Pathomechanics: As impingement is part of the painful arc syndrome, due to the trapping of the soft tissues, a drop in torque is evident in the painful range, although the rest of the range is normal.

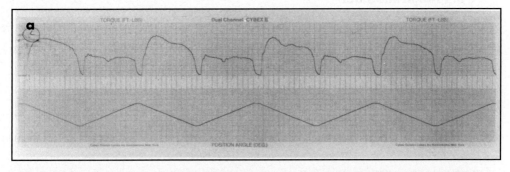

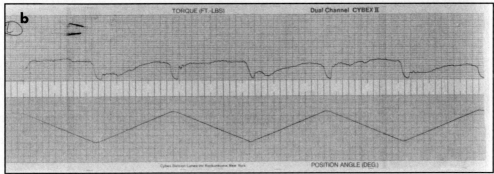

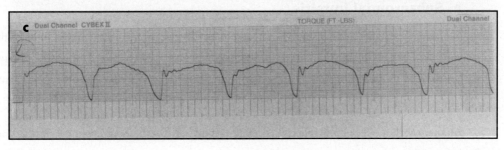

Figure 5-18 a) A sharp and significant drop at the mid-range of abduction and adduction. b) A drop at the initial range of flexion. c) An average peak torque curve of shoulder internal/external rotation testing.

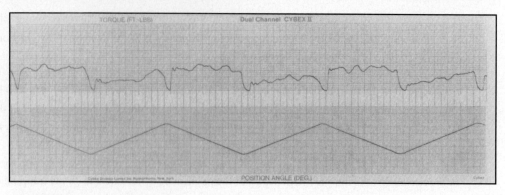

Figure 5-19 A curve from a patient with a frozen shoulder.

b. Frozen shoulder

Definition: Also known as adhesive capsulitis, the term frozen shoulder identifies glenohumeral joint pain and stiffness that cannot be explained by joint incongruity. The restriction of the passive range of motion is the hallmark of this condition.

Characteristics (Figure 5-19):

1) PT tends to be low, and sometimes it is impossible to test the patient because of the pain;

2) It is often difficult to reproduce test curves;

3) The curves produced tend to be very shaky; and

4) The ROM is very limited.

Pathomechanics: Pain inhibition, especially at the extremes of the ROM, makes force generation difficult. This pain affects the reproducibility, and thus the reliability, of the measured PT.

c. Subacromial bursitis

Definition: A bursa lies between the supraspinatus muscle and the acromion process of the scapula. Swelling of the bursa is due to inflammation, which is often caused by a fall or a blow to the shoulder. Sometimes, it can be caused by supraspinatus tendon rupture, which bleeds into the bursa causing inflammation (Peterson and Renström 1986).

Characteristics: The curve shape is similar to that seen with shoulder impingement, but bursitis exhibits a less sharp and a heavier depression. Generally, PT is lower in bursitis than in impingement (Figure 5-20).

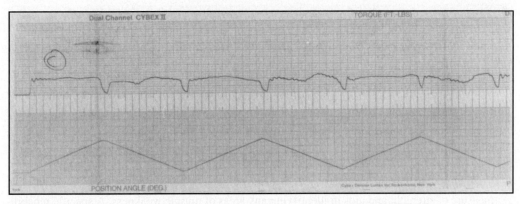

Figure 5-20 A curve produced by a patient with subacromial bursitis. Depressions at mid-range are less sharp but heavier.

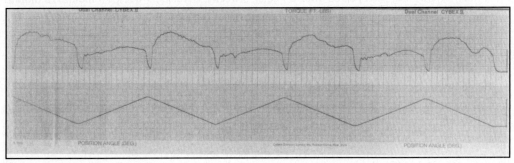

Figure 5-21 A curve produced by a patient with subscapular tendinitis. The depressions occur during the later test repetitions.

Pathomechanics: The pathomechanics is similar to the impingement syndrome, but, due to the persistent pain, PT is generally lower on the affected side.

d. Tendinitis of the subscapularis

Definition: The subscapularis muscle originates on the inner surface of the scapula and inserts into the anterior aspect of the head of humerus. It is the most important internal rotator of the shoulder of the upper arm. Inflammation of the subscapularis tendon is common in throwers, pitchers and racket sport players who involve overhead play (Peterson and Renström 1986).

Characteristics: The torque curve is similar to that seen with bursitis, but, in tendinitis, a dramatic drop in PT is common, often occurring during later test repetitions. This drop is typically seen in both of the opposing muscle groups. Despite the drop, the shape of the curve may be maintained (Figure 5-21).

Pathomechanics: The pathomechanics is similar to that seen with bursitis and consists of impaired power of the arm movements involving inward rotation. Tendonitis causes pain later in the movement instead.

F. Use of isokinetics in injury assessment and rehabilitation

1. Basic principles of assessment and rehabilitation

Isokinetic training can start as soon as CPM is indicated. This should be done in gravity eliminated planes of movements when the involved muscle is above grade 2 according to the MRC muscle grading. When the limb is able to perform a free active movement, gravity resisted exercise can also be included. The main areas of muscle training include strength, power, work and endurance.

An initial isokinetic test determines the status of a given muscle group, providing a baseline measure of strength, and aids in identifying any areas of muscle weakness. A specific rehabilitation program can then be designed. Evaluation of progress should be continuous. After the initial test, this may be repeated after 2 weeks, 3 weeks, 6 weeks, 9 weeks, 3 months, 6 months and then every 6 months. The rehabilitation program is adjusted according to subsequent test results.

In the following synopsis, some basic principles of injury diagnosis and rehabilitation, utilizing isokinetics, will be presented.

Diagnosis	Bilateral comparisons, cross-sectional data comparison, longitudinal progress reports and torque curves.
Rehabilitation	Muscle strengthening
	Joint mobility (CPM)
	Strength assessment
Stage I	Control of signs and symptoms
	Rest
Stage II	Prevention of complications:
	Muscle atrophy
	Joint stiffness
	Control of signs and symptoms
Stage III	Conditioning :
	Muscle strengthening
	Increase joint mobility
	Increase flexibility
	Coordination training
	Proprioception training
Stage IV	Prevention of recurrence :
	Maintain muscle characteristics
	Maintain joint characteristics
	Maintain functional abilities

Isokinetics is progressively introduced from Stage II onward. Its contribution increases during Stages III and IV.

The primary goal of rehabilitation is to facilitate the patient's full return to normal activity at the pre-injury level as quickly as possible. With athletes, the medical team has to be knowledgeable about the sport, athletes, position in the team, and the psychological impact of the injury to the athlete in order to provide effective and appropriate treatment.

The principles of isokinetic muscle training are described in the following diagram:

Principles of isokinetic training

Start training only when the limb is able to do free movement, or work against gravity

Start with a fast speed (180°/s), and progress by reducing speed

⬇

Control ROM

⬇

Exercise should be painfree

⬇

Training should be suspended if adverse effects emerge, such as effusion, pain, joint swelling, limb swelling, paresthesia

DO NOT OVERTRAIN

Dvir (1995) highlights the fact that protocols and procedures for isokinetic muscle function testing are relatively well established, while its clinical role in muscle conditioning is still less well understood. There are no hard and fast rules regarding appropriate protocols for the rehabilitation of common injuries.

In the following paragraphs, we will describe assessment and rehabilitation protocols used in our laboratory. Most of our research experience is related to the assessment and rehabilitation of the knee, ankle and the trunk, but studies are underway on the shoulder joint. We will therefore describe our own work in some details, while the rehabilitation of other joints and muscle groups, such as the hip, elbow and wrist, for which we have only limited experience, will be covered under the section on localized muscle weakness. This information is based on the work of other authors. At the end of the section, a synopsis of testing protocols for the major joints, including the hip, elbow and wrist will be provided.

2. Assessment and rehabilitation of the knee joint
a. Anterior cruciate ligament deficiency

Anterior cruciate ligament injuries (Figure 5-22) in athletes are common (Maffulli et al 1993). They are always serious and their rehabilitation is long. Yet, the management of ACLI remains controversial. An untreated ACL tear may result in deterioration of knee function with the development of rotatory instability, meniscal tears, progressive degeneration of articular cartilage, and eventually, post-traumatic arthritis (Sandberg and Balkfors 1988, Giove et al 1983, McDaniel and Dameron 1983). Some authors believe that primary repair and/or reconstruction are necessary for stability and normal function (Marshall and Rubin 1977, O'Donoghue 1973), while others claim good results with conservative treatment (Giove et al 1983, Paulos et al 1981, Chick and Jackson 1978). Although an ACL tear tends to be associated with a greater degree of atrophy in the quadriceps muscle group than, for example, a medial collateral ligament tear, strengthening of the hamstrings muscles has been shown to be important in improving the function of an ACL deficient knee (Li et al 1996). Such an increase in the strength of the hamstrings may reduce the likelihood of antero-lateral subluxation of the tibia (Kannus 1988).

The next part will describe our work regarding the rehabilitation of the ACLI knee. Forty-six recreational athletes had an ACL tear confirmed clinically (Figure 5-23) and arthroscopically. Isokinetic testing of the knee extensors and flexors, using the Cybex II+, was performed 2 weeks after arthroscopy. According to the isokinetic test results, an individual training program was designed. Pain relief and control of swelling were achieved using local ice application and interferential therapy.

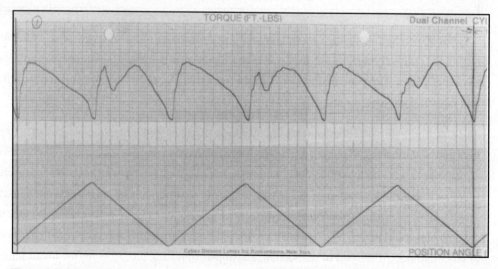

Figure 5-22 The use of isokinetic test results in injury diagnosis and rehabilitation.

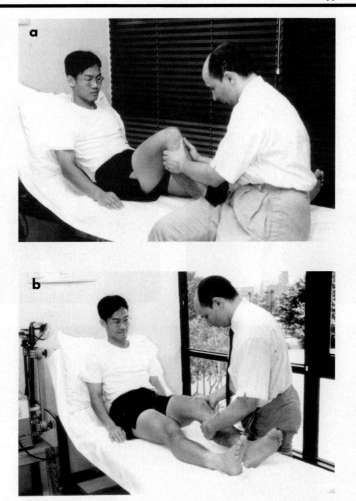

Figure 5-23 a) and b) Examination of the knee joint — the anterior drawer's test for ACL insufficiency.

Aim: Isokinetic training aimed at strengthening the quadriceps and hamstrings muscle groups, establishing a H:Q ratio approaching one on the injured side, and minimizing contralateral strength discrepancies to within 15%. The training program was adjusted individually according to each athlete's progress.

b. Testing protocol for the ACLI knee

Clinical ability test: This was assessed using a modified Cincinnati rating scale (Li et al 1996).

General warm-up: A 5-minute warm-up including rhythmic activity was performed, followed by a quadriceps and a hamstrings stretch (Figure 5-24). Warm-up needs to be modified depending on injury.

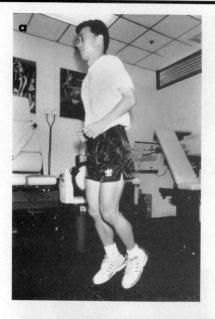
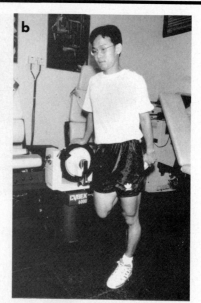
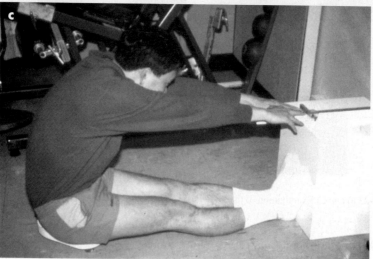

Figure 5-24 a) An athlete warming up prior to a knee test. b) A quadriceps stretch. c) A hamstrings stretch.

Joint alignment: All tests were done in a seated position. The hip and the trunk were positioned at an angle of 110° (Figure 5-25).

Stabilization: A velcro strap was fastened at the waist, across the trunk and across the thighs (Figure 5-26).

Variables assessed: Peak torque, peak torque to weight ratio, peak torque acceleration energy, average power, endurance ratio, and concentric/eccentric ratio were included.

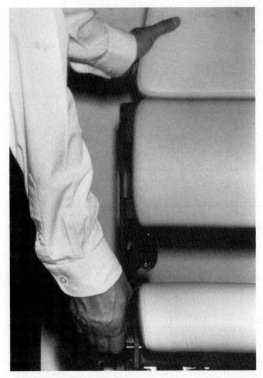

Figure 5-25 Tilting the back support at an angle with the seat so that when the patient is seated, the hip and trunk will make an angle between 100° and 110°.

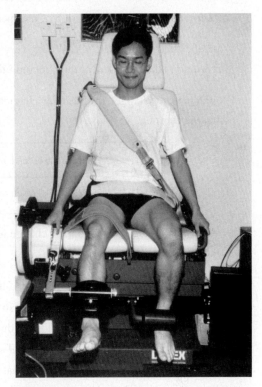

Figure 5-26 Patient is well strapped and supported for stability.

Velocity: Velocities used were 60°/s and 180°/s.

Test specific warm-up: Five repetitions were performed before each test movement and each speed.

Repetitions and sets: PT was measured from five maximal contractions at 60°/s. Endurance was measured from twenty-five contractions at 180°/s. A one-minute rest period was allowed between the speeds and 5 minutes between the limbs.

Encouragement given: Verbal encouragement was given throughout the test.

Test order : The unaffected side was tested first.

c. ACL tear: rehabilitation program

Training: Training for PT development of the knee flexor/extensor muscles was done at 60°/s, including five repetitions per set, with 5 to 10 seconds between the sets. Training for endurance was done at 180°/s, including twenty to fifty repetitions per set, with 20 to 30 seconds between the sets.

Duration: Ten minutes at each of the speeds, three times per week for 6 weeks.

If the quadriceps group was already very strong, little specific strengthening was needed, as this would make it harder for the H:Q ratio to approach one.

Percentage changes in muscular characteristics and in functional ability were calculated using the formula:

$$\frac{\text{Result of the second test} - \text{Result of the first test}}{\text{Result of the first test}} \times 100\%$$

The functional score percentage change was correlated to the percentage change in different isokinetic muscle strength variables.

Outcome: Evaluation of the outcome of this training regimen revealed that the H:Q ratio, at 30° flexion at 180°/s, was closely related to the improvement in the functional score. All the characteristics, including PT, AP, TW, endurance and PKTAE of the hamstrings group were significantly associated with the functional score, while the quadriceps muscle characteristics were not. The results strongly suggested that increasing the H:Q ratio at high angular velocities will result in a significant improvement in the functional ability of an ACL deficient knee. Thus, in the short-term, strengthening of the hamstrings group should be prominent in the rehabilitation process. Training should be specific and we advocate incorporating PT, power, PKTAE and endurance training. Although isokinetic quadriceps muscle characteristics were not found to be associated with the functional ability of the ACL-deficient knee, Li et al (1996) and Kannus (1988) emphasized the importance of maintaining a minimum quadriceps strength of 85% of that of the uninjured knee. The quadriceps tends to be more prone to atrophy than the hamstrings in ACL injured knees (Kannus 1988, Vegso et al 1985), and should be specifically trained after knee injury.

The use of a shin pad: Compressive and shear forces are produced at the knee joint during knee extension. The quadriceps shifts the proximal tibia forward creating an excessive stress on the anterior cruciate deficient knee. In 1982, Johnson introduced the "antishear device" (Cybex, Division of Lumex, Ronkonkoma, New York, USA) for the rehabilitation of knee injuries. The Johnson antishear device was designed to decrease anterior translational force during knee extension, preventing further damage to the joint. The effectiveness of the device has been confirmed by Timm (1986). Importantly, torque production has been reported to be lower when using the antishear device. Nisell et al (1989) found that isokinetic torque was lower when the resistance pad was placed more proximally. Li et al (1993) reported that the Johnson antishear device produced a significantly different value for knee extension in terms of PT, AW and AP at all speeds except medium speed PT, whereas no significant differences in knee flexion were found, except for the slow speed AW. Further, all the mean values from the standard shin pad were greater than with the Johnson antishear device. The difference between flexion and extension torques produced with the two devices is considered to be a result of the subject's unfamiliarity, at least when the pad is placed near the knee joint. Higher resistance forces may induce subliminal pain, or other inhibiting influences from cutaneous and/or periosteal mechanoreceptor afferent nerves (Nisell et al 1989). Also, the higher resistance force may influence the relative position of the tibia to the femur, and thus shorten the patella tendon moment arm. In summary, the same shin pad should be used to compare torque values between injured and uninjured limbs, and in subsequent tests.

3. Assessment and rehabilitation of the ankle joint

In the following paragraphs, assessment and rehabilitation procedures for ankle inversion injury will be presented. The data were collected as a part of a research project between The Chinese University of Hong Kong and the Hong Kong Sports Institute (HKSI) (Yeung et al 1992).

Ankle sprain is a common traumatic injury in sport, and often regarded as trivial (Korkia et al 1994, Lewin 1989, Smith and Reischl 1986, Cetti et al 1982,), leading to residual symptoms and recurrent sprains. This is often the result of neglect, lack of medical involvement and inadequate rehabilitation (Smith and Reischl 1986). A number of factors contribute to the recurrence of ankle sprains, including muscle weakness around the ankle, decreased proprioception, tightness in the calf muscles and joint laxity (Lindenfeld 1988, Kaumeyer and Malone 1980,). A local survey of sports injuries between 1988 and 1989 revealed that 15% of all sports injuries sustained were ankle sprains. An epidemiologic survey of 380 athletes with previous history of ankle sprains was then conducted between 1990 and 1991 among Hong Kong Chinese athletes taking part in a variety of sports (Yeung et al 1994). Seventy-one percent of the respondents were men, and 29% were women. A total of 563 sprained ankles were recorded. An injury only to the dominant side was two point four times greater than injury only to the non-dominant side. Typically, injury occurred during the middle or latter part of the sports session. There was a trend toward an increase in complaints of residual symptoms, such as instability, chronic swelling, pain, weakness, stiffness and crepitus, with an increased number of ankle sprains sustained.

Thirty-one subjects, 25 men and 6 women (25.3±5.5 years of age) participating in different sports and with history of unilateral recurrent ankle inversion sprain participated in the rehabilitation study. Fifty non-injured subjects, 25 men and 25 women in their mid-twenties, were also tested to obtain normative data. The Cybex II+ isokinetic dynamometer was used for all tests.

Aim: The aim of the investigation was to obtain an objective and comprehensive evaluation of ankle characteristics following recurrent ankle sprains, to suggest a method for evaluating functional capabilities of the sprained ankle, and to develop an effective rehabilitation program for such an injury.

a. Ankle sprain: assessment

Each subject came to the HKSI on two separate occasions to test two different ankle movements. During the first session, ankle dorsiflexion/plantarflexion (DF/PF) was determined. The second session involved the testing of ankle eversion/inversion (EV/IV). Subjects were asked to wear unrestrictive clothing and sports shoes.

b. Test procedure for ankle sprain

Clinical ability test: 1) A manual anterior drawer test (Figure 5-27) was performed by a sports physician. Twelve ankles demonstrated a positive anterior drawer test in the injured ankles, while 19 showed no anterior subluxation; 2) both active and passive ankle dorsiflexion ROM were significantly decreased in the injured ankles; and 3) ankle functional rating scale was 82.3±8.6 points out of 100. None scored 100 in the initial test. There is no specific method for establishing an exact diagnosis and for grading ankle sprain. The subject's own description of the injury was relied upon and thus it was difficult to ascertain whether a partial or complete tear had occurred. The severity of injuries may have varied, affecting subsequent muscle strength and functional score measurements.

General warm-up: Before each session, subjects were required to perform 10 minutes of cycling on a Monark cycle ergometer, set at one Watts per kilogram per body weight. This was followed by 5 minutes of stretching of the lower limbs.

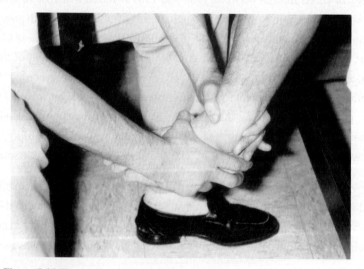

Figure 5-27 The anterior drawer test of the ankle joint

Joint alignment: 1) Ankle DF/PF was measured in a prone position, with the knees extended. The foot was fixed into a PF/DF foot-plate. The subject was positioned so that the hip was internally rotated to approximately 16°. The axis of the movement at the talocrural joint was then aligned with the axis of the dynamometer. The foot was placed flat on the foot-plate to ensure a neutral position (ie, neither inverted nor everted) (Figure 5-28); and 2) ankle EV/IV was measured in a supine position with the upper body exercise table seat in its highest position. The dynamometer head was tilted back 55°. The ankle was placed on the IV/EV plate. The subject was positioned so that the ankle was in a complete neutral position (Figure 5-29), determined by palpation, so that the head of talus was in a neutral position.

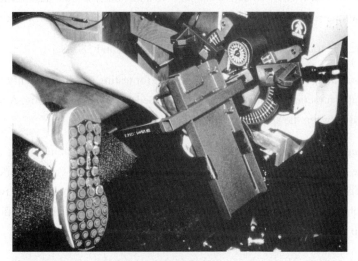

Figure 5-28 The ankle dorsiflexion/plantarflexion foot-plate.

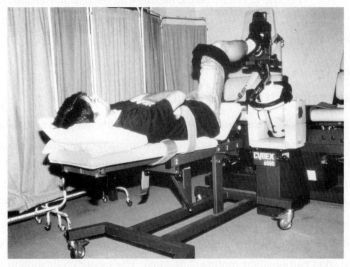

Figure 5-29 The ankle is at its neutral position ready for an ankle inversion/eversion test.

Stabilization: 1) DF/PF: The pelvic strap was used to stabilize the upper leg just above the knees. An additional torso strap was used to immobilize the upper trunk; and 2) IV/EV: The knee of the tested ankle was stabilized with the inversion/eversion input adaptor, and flexed between 30° and 75°. The dynamometer axis transected the superior edge of the lateral malleolus. Both alignment and stabilization were set according to the Cybex handbook, with the exception of two stoppers, which were placed to limit the ROM of inversion and eversion, and to prevent excessive tibial rotational movement, especially during the endurance test. The pelvis was stabilized with the pelvic strap.

Variables assessed: ROM of active and passive ankle dorsiflexion, peak torque, peak torque to weight ratio, average power, peak torque acceleration energy and total work were assessed.

Velocity: The training velocities employed were 60°/s and 180°/s.

Repetitions and sets: Five repetitions were used for testing PT, while twenty-five repetitions of reciprocal contractions at maximal force were used for endurance testing. A one-minute rest was allowed between the speeds and 5 minutes between the limbs.

Encouragement given: Subjects were instructed to exert maximum effort throughout the test. For the PT test at 60°/s, no verbal encouragement was given. For the work test at 180°/s, subjects were instructed to exert maximum force throughout the whole test of twenty-five repetitions. Subjects were encouraged twice, at the tenth and twentieth repetitions, by saying "good, keep going".

Warm-up and test: Three submaximal and three maximal contractions were used as a warm-up on the machine. This also familiarized the patient with the machine and the test speeds to be used. A one-minute rest interval was given between the warm-ups and the actual test, and between the two different speeds.

Test order: The ankle of the non-dominant leg was tested first.

c. Ankle rehabilitation program

Half of the subjects from the injury group were randomly assigned to the isokinetic training group while the other half served as controls. The training group underwent isokinetic training for ankle DF/PF and ankle IV/EV. Ankle DF/PF was completed first, followed by IV/EV exercise. Velocity spectrum training was employed, from 60°/s up to 240°/s, at 60°/s intervals (ie, 60°/s, 120°/s, 180°/s, 240°/s, 180°/s, 120°/s, 60°/s). Ten repetitions at each training speed were performed in a pyramid fashion. One-minute rest was allowed between the speeds and 30 minutes between DF/PF and IV/EV. Training took place three times per week for 6 weeks and daily activities and sport participation continued as usual. The second evaluation of muscle strength was done 8 to 10 weeks after the first evaluation.

Outcome: The mean PT of ankle PF/DF and IV/EV were generally lower than those of the uninjured side when measured at 60°/s and 180°/s.

The mean increases (%) in PT, AP, TW and PKTAE after 6 weeks of training are shown in Table 5-2.

PT (60°/s)	PT (180°/s)	AP	PKTAE	TW
PF: 13.5	23.0 *	32.2 *	21.1 *	34.5 *
DF: 15.0	14.3 *	44.3 *	27.0 *	23.5 *
EV: 44.6 *	28.4*	44.3 *	40.2 *	44.4 *
IV : 15.4	44.6 *	55.2*	33.4 *	55.5 *

Note: PT=Peak torque, AP=Average power, PKTAE=Peak torque acceleration energy, TW=Total work, PF=Plantarflexion, DF=Dorsiflexion, EV=Eversion and IV=Inversion.
* statistically significant difference at 5% level.

Table 5-2 Mean increases (%) in peak torque, average power, total work done and peak torque acceleration energy in ankle dorsiflexion/plantarflexion and eversion/inversion after 6 weeks of training (n=14).

The functional score of the injured ankle in the second test for the exercise group increased from 80.7±10.2 to 90.3±7.1 (p<0.05), while no significant changes were detected in the control group (83.8±6.2 and 84.3±5.4).

Sprains of the dominant ankle appeared to induce greater generalized muscle weakening than injury to the non-dominant ankle. A possible explanation is that the dominant leg was usually the leading leg, and would have been activated more in explosive and strenuous activities, such as jumping, hopping and kicking. Further, injury to the dominant ankle would require a longer rest period before returning to vigorous activities. A shorter rest period would result in a lesser degree of disuse muscle atrophy and subsequent weakness. Injured ankles had consistently lower ROM in active and passive DF, whereas no such discrepancy was measured for DF in the control group. This was suggested to be an indication of calf muscle tightness after inversion ankle sprain. Tight calf muscles have been linked with an increased risk of sustaining a recurrent ankle sprain (Walsh and Blackburn 1977). Weaknesses in ankle EV and DF were often described as the underlying cause for recurrent ankle inversion sprains. The role of these muscles is to provide dynamic support to the lateral ligaments for maintaining stability of the ankle joint and for counteracting the inversion force in an ankle sprain (Diamond 1989, Garn and Newton 1988). Pain and immobility after injury lead to muscle weakness, followed by secondary muscle atrophy, easily causing recurrent injury (Grace 1984). Therefore, strengthening of an injured ankle is essential for breaking such a vicious circle of pain and disuse.

This investigation demonstrated substantial improvements in muscle strength characteristics, such as torque, power, endurance and acceleration in sprained ankles, trained with isokinetics three times a week for 6 weeks. Yet, only 2 of the 16 subjects who underwent isokinetic training recovered fully, ie, to 100 points in the functional score from their ankle injury. Six weeks may not be enough to achieve full recovery.

4. Assessment and rehabilitation of the trunk

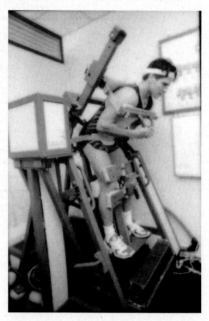

Information regarding isokinetic rehabilitation of the trunk is scarce. As we have used isokinetics in rehabilitation of back problems for the past 3 years, we will present some research data on trunk flexion/extension measures with athletes, and then describe our rehabilitation protocol. The effectiveness of this protocol has not been formally tested, however (Figure 5-30).

The trunk and the back are complex structures which contribute to performance in most daily and sporting activities. In many sports, such as tennis, squash, and discus throwing the back is used to initiate many movements and to perform them to the full. Trunk muscle strength is considered of vital importance in protecting the spine against back strains (Morris et al 1961). Muscle strength in the trunk is required to stabilize the lower spinal segments and to distribute

Figure 5-30 Isokinetic trunk flexion/extension testing using the TEF unit.

forces throughout the entire abdominal and thoracic cavities. In sporting actions, abdominal and oblique muscles strength is needed to provide stability, to allow effective bending, pulling and twisting (Pauletto 1991), and to prevent injury (Broccoletti 1981). In swimming, for instance, balance and power are primarily derived from the back musculature. Strokes such as the butterfly utilize mainly back muscles (Broccoletti 1981).

a. Low back pain

Low back pain causes a loss of 217 million work days a year in USA (Frymoer et al 1983), and 17% of all adults in USA report some back symptoms at some point during their lives (Krazier et al 1984). We still do not know, however, why many patients suffer from low back pain, how exactly it develops, what its causes are, and who is at risk (D'Orazio 1993). Weakness in the abdominal muscles in patients with low back pain is frequently reported (Hause et al 1980) and an evaluation of 4,000 cases of low back pain demonstrated that some abdominal muscle weaknesses were present (Smidt et al 1980). Larson (1961) and Klausen (1965) highlighted the need for balanced strength between the long flexors and extensors in the prevention

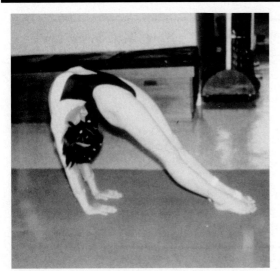

Figure 5-31 Gymnasts putting a lot of stress to their back often cause low back pain.

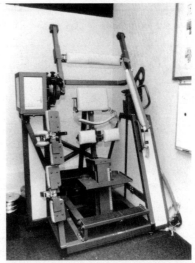

Figure 5-32 The Cybex Trunk Extension and Flexion Unit.

of low back dysfunction. A significant relationship was found between the strength levels of abdominal muscles and back muscles, and the ratio of the two was less than one in most of the patients studied by Hause et al (1980). They also suggested that patients with strong abdominal muscles also tended to have strong back muscles. Further, Addison and Schultz (1980) reported a smaller ratio of back extension to flexion in patients with back pain than in normal subjects (Figure 5-31).

b. Isokinetic testing of the trunk

In the following paragraphs, testing the trunk and back muscles for the assessment of abnormalities will be described.

Aim: The aim of the study was twofold. 1) To determine the trunk muscle characteristics of elite Hong Kong male athletes from a variety of sports, and to compare these data to sedentary subjects of the same age; 2) to ascertain whether trunk muscle characteristics differ between individuals engaged in different sports.

Thirty-five athletes who were Hong Kong national team members in badminton, canoeing, cycling, rowing and squash participated in the study. Fifty-two sedentary males of the same age served as controls. Physical characteristics and sports background of the subjects is presented in Table 5-3. Individuals with known cardiovascular, neuromuscular, and muscular problems were excluded from the study. Individuals who had undergone spinal surgery or had been bedridden for one day or more in the past three years were excluded from the study. All tests were performed using the Cybex Trunk Extension/Flexion Testing and Rehabilitation Unit (TEF)(Figure 5-32).

Subject groups	Age (yrs)	Height(cm)	Weight (kg)	%Body fat	Lean weight (kg)
Non-athletic (n=52)	22.0 (2.6)	171.0 (5.2)	61.3 (8.5)	9.9 (6.0)	55.1 (5.6)
Badminton (n=5)	22.8 (1.3)	172.8 (6.8)	62.0 (3.7)	4.0 (0.4)	59.6 (3.7)
Squash (n=7)	21.3 (2.0)	173.0 (3.8)	67.9 (9.9)	7.1 (5.4)	62.6 (5.7)
Cycling (n=7)	22.7 (2.7)	172.1 (2.8)	63.1 (4.6)	5.3 (0.7)	59.8 (4.0)
Rowing (n=7)	22.6 (5.8)	175.6 (3.1)	71.6 (2.2)	6.9 (2.0)	66.4 (3.0)
Canoeing(n=9)	23.1 (6.1)	172.1 (3.6)	69.0 (7.5)	7.9 (3.5)	63.2 (5.0)

Table 5-3 Physical characteristics of athletic and non-athletic subjects (mean and standard deviation).

c. Isokinetic testing protocol for the trunk and the back

Warm-up: A 10-minute warm-up including cycling on a Monark cycle ergometer at 60rpm at one watt per kilogram of body weight. This was followed by 10-minute of stretching, with emphasis on trunk muscles.

Joint alignment: The axis of the dynamometer was centered at the L5-S1 intervertebral segment. The starting posture for testing was located at the biomechanically-derived anatomical zero (Figure 5-33).

Stabilization: The lower body was stabilized in a slightly bent-knee position by tibial, popliteal and thigh pads (Figure 5-34), and a pelvic belt. The shoulder girdle complex was stabilized to minimize the potential contribution of upper extremity muscle groups to the lumbar and lower extremity muscle performance efforts (Figure 5-35).

Variables assessed: The variables assessed included peak torque, peak torque to body weight, work, total work and agonist/antagonist muscle group ratios.

Test velocity: The velocities employed were 60°/s, 90°/s and 120°/s.

Repetitions and sets: Four maximal flexion/extension repetitions were done at 60°/s and 90°/s, and twenty repetitions at 120°/s. There was a 30-second rest period between maximum contractions at the different testing speeds.

Range of motion: The motion arc used was 15° to 60° from a vertical starting point, flexion from vertical to a position of 60° from vertical, and extension was 60° from vertical to 15° from the vertical (ie, moving back).

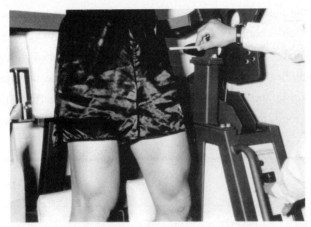

Figure 5-33 Aligning the back movement axis at the L5-S1 level and the axis of the dynamometer for the trunk flexion/extension test.

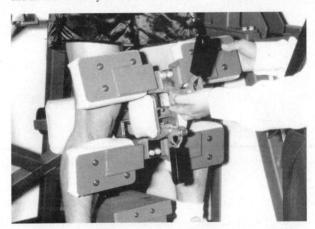

Figure 5-34 Insertion of the shin and thigh pad to support the knee and to maintain the knee in a slightly flexed position.

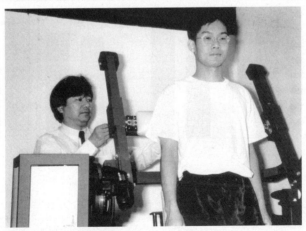

Figure 5-35 Stabilizing the shoulder girdle complex.

Results: In the non-athletic group, trunk extension performance was significantly better than flexion. A drop in both extension and flexion as a result of increasing test speed could be expected. Total body weight and lean body weight were associated with greater PT performance in both trunk flexion and extension. The athletic group generated greater values than the non-athletic group in almost all measures. Table 5-4 shows the PT values generated by the different sports groups for flexion and extension at 60°/s, 90°/s and 120°/s.

Subject groups	Flex 60°/s	Flex 90°/s	Flex 120°/s	Ext 60°/s	Ext 90°/s	Ext 120°/s
Non-athletic	206 (42)	195 (37)	187 (33)	286 (67)	263 (58)	235 (55)
Badminton	249 (26)	248 (24)	243 (22)	368 (34)	392 (37)	381 (41)
Squash	256 (38)	260 (42)	249 (35)	352 (64)	348 (53)	320 (42)
Cycling	216 (29)	216 (25)	211 (22)	329 (50)	321 (44)	292 (45)
Rowing	287 (48)	278 (47)	262 (41)	389 (82)	367 (79)	356 (53)
Canoeing	304 (30)	294 (29)	284 (26)	350 (47)	337 (42)	319 (39)

Table 5-4 Peak torque (Nm) results for the different sports groups (mean and standard deviation).

Badminton players scored highest in trunk extension, with the exception of PT at 60°/s, and absolute work and total work at 120°/s. Badminton players were significantly better than the canoeists and cyclists in relative measures, which accounted for body weight. This probably

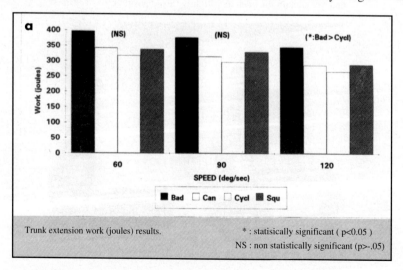

Trunk extension work (joules) results.

* : statisically significant (p<0.05)
NS : non statistically significant (p>-.05)

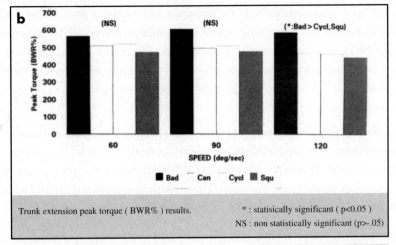

Trunk extension peak torque (BWR%) results.   * : statisically significant (p<0.05)
NS : non statistically significant (p>-.05)

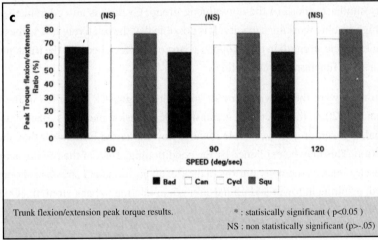

Trunk flexion/extension peak torque results.   * : statisically significant (p<0.05)
NS : non statistically significant (p>-.05)

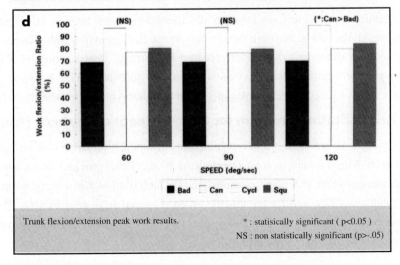

Trunk flexion/extension peak work results.   * : statisically significant (p<0.05)
NS : non statistically significant (p>-.05)

Figure 5-36 a) to d) The results of an isokinetic trunk test in different athletic groups.

reflects the need to extend the body for smashing and overhead play. Under normal circumstances, PT declines with increasing speed. In badminton players, the reverse was observed. This may be in response to the functional demands of the game, resulting in specific neuromuscular adaptations. Badminton players, as a group, scored better at higher speeds in both extension and flexion tests. For the trunk flexion/extension PT and work ratios, badminton players scored lowest (Figure 5-36).

The squash players produced lower scores than badminton players and rowers in trunk extension, and lower than the canoeists and rowers in the flexion test. Nevertheless, the results obtained were good. This may be explained by the demands of the sport, which stresses spinal flexion and rotation, and trunk extension. The trunk flexion/extension PT and work ratios were between 74% and 82%, a range similar to that of the rowers.

Cyclists scored lower, in all measures, compared to the other sports groups. Their results were very similar to those of the non-athletic group. Cycling is an endurance sport which requires a high aerobic working capacity. It is possible that the relatively low values demonstrated in the trunk muscle strength in this group is a carryover effect, because the trunk muscles mainly perform a static function during cycling.

The rowers were the heaviest group, and scored highest PT at 60°/s in the trunk flexion movement. At 120°/s, they recorded greatest trunk extension measures. Back extensor strength is essential in generating power while rowing. Rowers scored little lower than the canoeists in trunk flexion. This may be explained by the conditioning effect of the rowing action, where the trunk muscles relax as the body returns to the flexed position, and stress on abdominal muscles is reduced, resulting in lower abdominal strength in relation to back strength. On average, they scored 75% in PT ratio and 77% in work ratio, which is slightly below the accepted range (80% to 90%).

The canoeists tended to score lower in all variables measured than the other groups. They were, however, the best in the trunk flexion movement. Because of the high values scored in the flexion test, the canoeists' values were greatest in the trunk flexion/extension PT and work ratios, at all speeds tested. Their flexion/extension ratio approached one. It appears that canoeists require such a ratio for the maintenance of an upright body position during pedaling.

d. Rehabilitation program for the treatment of low back pain

Information on isokinetic trunk rehabilitation is limited. Normative data on trunk flexion/extension for Asians are also scarce. The study by Wong (1994) provides useful normative data for both sedentary and athletic populations. The PT ratio of trunk flexion/extension for normal young adults was 72% and for the athletic group it ranged from 66% to 88%. The accepted range has been set between 80% and 90%. These values can be used as guidelines on isokinetic trunk rehabilitation of back conditions.

Isokinetic rehabilitation starts when symptoms have subsided. At this stage, the patient should only have mild back pain, limited trunk movement, and, most prominently, weak muscle strength. Rehabilitation aims at controlling signs and symptoms, if any, and strengthening the trunk muscles by exercise against one's own body weight. The rehabilitation protocol outlined below is the one we have used since 1991 with good results in the routine rehabilitation of low back pain.

e. Rehabilitation protocol for low back pain

Stage I

1) Daily static back exercises such as pressing the back against a firm mattress, followed by arching of the back;

2) Isokinetic trunk exercises are performed at mid-ROM (or painfree range). Five sets of six repetitions of flexion and extension at 120°/s using the TEF unit three times a week;

3) Rest and ice treatment after exercise.

Stage II

When signs and symptoms are controlled, progressive isokinetic trunk exercise can commence. The aim is to further strengthen the trunk muscles. The protocol is as follows:

1) Isokinetic trunk exercises performed at a larger range (eg, 15° extension and 45° flexion). Five sets of six repetitions of flexion and extension at 120°/s followed by five sets of six repetitions at 90°/s, with 15 to 20 seconds rest between the sets. Exercises to be done daily;

2) If no complications or adverse effects are experienced, progress by performing five sets of six repetitions at 60°/s, with 15 to 20 seconds rest between the sets;

3) For further progress at this stage, increase the number of repetitions and encourage the patient to work harder;

4) Gentle flexibility, coordination and balance training;

5) Ice therapy if required;

6) Patient education on back care.

Stage III

When the patient is able to perform daily activities without too much difficulty, and has no adverse effects after isokinetic training, an isokinetic trunk test to assess the muscle status can be performed. Design a protocol in accordance to the test results, following the guidelines given above. In addition, general functional and sport-specific exercise may begin.

1) Isokinetic trunk exercise performed at full range daily;

2) Strength training as before at all speeds. Double the number of repetitions and exercise for 20 minutes. Add endurance training at 120°/s. Do twenty to thirty repetitions with 20 to 30 seconds rest in between the sets for 5 to 10 minutes;

3) Fast walking and running (with good shock absorbing shoes);

4) Start light sporting activity of patient's own choice;

5) Continue flexibility training;

6) Under great care, teach the patient to lift light objects.

Stage IV

When the patient is at the final stages of rehabilitation, the main aim is to ensure that the patient is exerting maximum effort. Isokinetic assessment is used to guide optimal loading for subsequent training program.

1) Isokinetic strength and endurance training using velocity spectrum training: 60°/s, 120°/s, 180°/s, six repetitions per set, with 15 to 20 seconds rest between the sets for strength. Endurance training: 120°/s and 180°/s, twenty to thirty repetitions per set with 20 to 30 seconds rest between the sets. Generally, training should involve as many repetitions as the patient can tolerate for 25 to 30 minutes, three to seven times per week;

2) Continue with flexibility, coordination and balance exercises;

3) Lifting objects, stair climbing, cutting, jumping and agility training may be incorporated;

4) Back to full sport participation.

When full rehabilitation is over, encourage the patient to maintain the achieved muscle strength to prevent recurrence of back pain. For maintenance of the acquired strength, at least weekly strength training is recommended. Encourage regular trunk muscle evaluation to detect any early signs of muscle weakness or imbalance.

5. Assessment and rehabilitation of shoulder impingement syndrome (bursitis, tendinitis and muscle impingement)

a. Testing protocol

For the three plane movements of shoulder abduction/adduction, flexion/extension, internal/external rotation at 0° abduction, select the plane causing least pain to the patient.

General warm-up: A 10-minute warm-up including rhythmic activity, followed by shoulder specific stretching (Figure 5-37).

Joint alignment and stabilization: According to the instructions given in the isokinetics testing handbook.

Range of movement: Set appropriate painfree range.

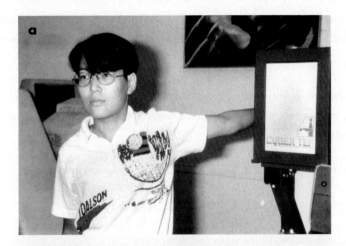

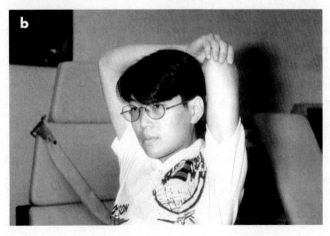

Figure 5-37 a) Shoulder abduction stretching. b) Shoulder external rotation stretching.

Variables assessed: Peak torque, work, peak torque acceleration energy, power and endurance ratio were assessed.

Velocity: Patients at 60°/s and 180°/s, and athletes up to 240°/s.

Test specific warm-up: Five repetitions before each test movement and each speed.

Repetitions and sets: Peak torque is measured from five maximal contractions at 60°/s and endurance from twenty-five contractions at 180°/s (240°/s for athletes) with less than a minute rest between the speeds, and 5 minutes between the limbs.

Test order: The unaffected side is tested first.

Shoulder impingement syndromes inflict pain within a specified arc, whereas the range outside this arc is painfree. Pain usually occurs around the acromion area. It is generally felt during overhead activities, such as smashing a tennis ball and stroking while swimming. The dual aim of rehabilitation is to allow inflammation to subside, and to strengthen the rotator cuff muscles.

Stage I

When the pain is still easily produced by simple overhead activities, exercise will involve gentle free movements without resistance, such as pointing, reaching or simply elevating the arm beyond 90°. Also:

1) Rest the involved shoulder, and control the signs and symptoms;

When pain begins to subside, commence isokinetic training.

2) Continue to control the signs and symptoms;

3) Choose the least painful movement plane: flexion/extension, abduction/adduction or the internal/external rotation of the shoulder for early rehabilitation;

4) Isokinetic exercise at 240°/s or even 300°/s at the beginning for 10 minutes, eight to ten repetitions per set with a 20-second rest between the sets. Repeat three to seven times per week;

5) Control the movement within the painfree range. Sometimes, in order to avoid the painful arc, this can be done as ranged movement of the same plane;

6) Start coordination and proprioceptive exercises;

7) Prescribe maintenance exercise for all-round muscle conditioning.

Stage III

When the pain is well under control and the patient is able to perform daily activities, such as dressing and undressing, combing the hair, using a knife and preparing food, start the next phase.

1) Progression can be made when no adverse effects from the previous exercise are experienced;

2) Progression has to be gradual;

3) Exercise progresses as follows:

a) Decrease speed from 180°/s to 60°/s, or 30°/s for athletes;

b) Increase the range (only within the painfree limit);

c) Increase the duration and/or frequency of exercise;

d) Incorporate other planes of shoulder motion.

4) Apply ice if the shoulder is swollen and hot after exercise;

5) Other upper limb exercises can be incorporated, for example, throwing objects, ironing clothes and wiping the floor. Light and gentle recreational activities, such as freestyle swimming and gentle racket games, may commence.

Stage IV

During the final stage of rehabilitation, all signs and symptoms should have disappeared. The patient can gradually return to their sport.

1) Progression of isokinetic training:

a) Decrease the speed of isokinetic exercise, concentrating on improving PT, endurance ratio (increase the number of repetitions) and explosive power;

b) Increase the duration of exercise while reducing its frequency;

c) Incorporate all planes of shoulder movement.

2) Incorporate all forms of functional exercise, such as lifting objects above the head, pouring water from a kettle/teapot and carrying a suitcase;

3) Continue with a variety of sports activities, except for those which require excessive shoulder movements producing pain.

Prevention of recurrence is the main concern after recovery.

6. Frozen shoulder

Testing protocol: The test is the same as for shoulder impingement. Emphasize the control of ROM and make sure that the patient is free of pain.

Frozen shoulder causes severe pain, limitation of movement and loss of function. Most orthopedic surgeons divide the rehabilitation process for this condition into three stages.

Stage I

During the first stage, pain is increasing. It is easily elicited by any shoulder movements or even at rest. This may be severe enough to awake the patient at night. Available ROM will decline, and the functional loss is obvious. The aim of management is to control pain and attempt to maintain the ROM.

1) Rest the shoulder and avoid excessive movements;

2) Control the pain by drug therapy and physiotherapy, including short-wave diathermy and interferential therapy.

Stage II

During the second stage, pain starts decreasing while the ROM still continues to decline. The aim of the treatment is to begin the restoration of lost function. This aim may be difficult to achieve because the ROM still continues to decrease, leaving little room for improvement.

1) Continue to control the pain;

2) Start pendulum exercises to the shoulder, including static and small movements within the painfree region to the deltoids, pectoralis major, and triceps muscles;

3) When pain is under better control, start shoulder exercises consisting of active and free movements;

4) It is safe to proceed onto isokinetic training only during a later phase. Exercise at 240°/s, five to eight repetitons per set, with 20 to 30 seconds rest between the sets. Train for 10 minutes, three to seven times per week. Apply mechanical blocks to limit excessive range. Start with internal and external rotation at 0°/s of shoulder abduction (Figures 5-38, 5-39).

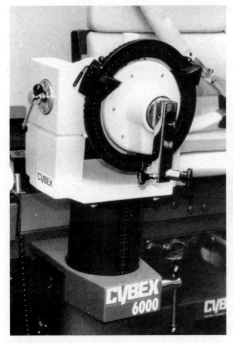

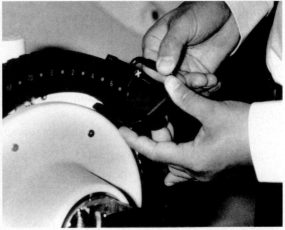

Figure 5-38 The "X" and "O" apparatus situated at the rim of the dynamometer are the mechanical blocks.

Figure 5-39 The mechanical block can be manually tightened and loosened by turning the lever arm, and can be manually slid along the rim of the dynamometer.

Stage III

The final stage usually begins several months after the onset of the condition. Pain continues to decrease, while ROM starts to increase. At this stage, treatment aims at restoring full function of the shoulder.

1) Continue isokinetic training:

    a) Internal/external rotation exercise at 0° abduction at 240°/s to 300°/s, ten repetitions per set, with 10 seconds rest between the sets, 5 to 10 minutes daily;

    b) The exercise must be done within the painfree range.

2) Progression is possible when no adverse effects from previous exercise is experienced;

3) Progression must be gradual;

4) Exercise progresses as follows:

    a) Decrease speed from 240°/s to 180°/s, and then to 60°/s;

    b) Increase the range (only within the painfree limit);

c) Increase the duration of exercise up to 20 to 30 minutes, and the frequency up to twice a day;

d) Perform exercises in other planes of shoulder motion, including flexion and extension, abduction and adduction.

5) Incorporate other forms of functional training, including ordinary daily tasks and recreational sport, as described for the shoulder impingement syndromes.

7. Assessment and rehabilitation of anterior knee pain (AKP)

Testing protocol: Isokinetic testing for AKP is the same as for ACLI.

AKP is due to many causes. Most often, it is caused by damage to the articular surface of the patella. In AKP, pain is experienced at the anterior aspect of the knee and behind the patella. Pain is generally produced by walking down a slope or descending stairs. The main aim of early rehabilitation is to shift the patella in relation to the anterior aspect of the femur. Other conditions for which the AKP rehabilitation program can be applied include patello-femoral joint pain, bursitis and patellar tendinitis.

Stage I

When pain is felt at rest or is easily produced by walking, the focus of treatment is to control signs and symptoms:

1) Rest the involved knee and bandage it if necessary;

2) Control the inflammation with ice and anti-inflammatory drugs.

When pain begins to subside, start isokinetic training of the hamstrings and quadriceps.

1) Continue to control signs and symptoms;

2) Identify the deficient side of patella and tape it away from the original position, if necessary;

3) Commence isokinetic exercise at 240°/s or even 300°/s, five sets of eight to ten repetitions with 20-second rest between the sets;

4) Control the movement within the painfree range, and use the mechanical blocks to limit the range as necessary:

a) For exercising the medial side, use 0° to 15° of knee flexion;

b) For exercising the lateral side, use 30° to 90° of knee flexion.

5) Exercise three to seven times per week, 10 minutes each time;

6) Apply ice after exercise;

7) Prescribe maintenance exercises for general muscle conditioning.

Stage II

When pain is well under control and the patient is able to walk without difficulty:

1) Progression can be made when no adverse effects from the previous exercise is experienced;

2) Progression must be gradual;

3) Exercise can progress in the following aspects:

a) Decrease speed;

b) Increase the ROM (only within the painfree limit);

c) Increase the duration and frequency of exercise;

d) Rely less on taping.

4) Apply ice after a training session;

5) Incorporate training for balance, coordination and proprioception;

6) Other forms of lower limb exercise may begin: walking down slopes, gentle recreational activities, such as swimming, cycling and jogging. Some forms of knee support may be required.

Stage III

During the final stages of rehabilitation, all signs and symptoms should have disappeared. Patients may gradually get more involved in their sport.

1) Progression of isokinetic training:

a) Lower speed isokinetic exercise, concentrate on high peak torque, endurance ratio and explosive power development;

b) Increase the duration of exercise, while decreasing its frequency, but not below three times per week;

c) Maintain appropriate ROM in the knee joint;

d) Commence eccentric isokinetic training at 60°/s for 10 minutes, including five to eight repetitions per set, with 10 to 15 seconds rest between the sets.

2) Start any form of sport activity, involving running, jumping, cutting and even stair climbing;

3) Begin a more aggressive balance training, coordination and agility exercise regime. Prevention of recurrence is the main concern after recovery. Patients with AKP are advised not to do prolonged kneeling, walking down stairs/slopes unnecessarily, perform weight-bearing deep knee bending, such as bunny hops, or ride a bicycle in a low seated position.

8. Assessment and rehabilitation of localized muscle weakness

The strength exerted by a given muscle or muscle group may decrease as a result of a number of conditions, such as traumatic injuries, surgery and prolonged immobilization. Once the underlying cause of muscle weakness has been identified, an appropriate strengthening regime can be prescribed.

Although hard scientific evidence is somewhat missing, it is logical to think that, if a muscle is deficient in strength, then at least some of its functions must be performed by surrounding muscles or muscle groups, which may thus be overloaded. Also, muscle exert a dampening effect of external traumas and serve as strain buffers to bone. Finally, if the contralateral muscle is normal, side-to-side imbalance may develop, and injuries may ensue.

In this respect, although the weakness of a muscle or muscle group can be an adaptive response to a specific sport, it makes sense to invest at least some of the training and rehabilitation program to minimize muscle weakness.

a. Isokinetic rehabilitation of localized muscle weakness

In acute conditions:

1) Control signs and symptoms;

2) Isokinetic exercise at 180°/s, three to five repetitions with 5 to 10 seconds rest between sets for 10 to 15 minutes each day;

3) Daily treatment is preferable;

4) Ice therapy after exercise is advisable;

5) Apply overload only when there are no adverse effects from the previous exercise session;

6) Progression must be gradual, and can be planned using the following criteria:

    a) Decrease speed;

    b) Increase the range (only within the painfree limit);

    c) Increase the duration and/or frequency of exercise.

7) Other forms of functional exercises, agility exercises and similar can be incorporated.

In chronic conditions:

1) Isokinetic exercise at 60°/s for 10 to 15 minutes, and 180°/s for 10 minutes, three times per week;

2) Ice therapy afterward;

3) Progress as in the acute conditions.

Synopsis of isokinetic testing protocols for the major joints

Note: rehabilitation of athletes will always involve a range of velocities. The tables give suggested minimums and maximums only.

Joint : Knee

Movement : Flexion and extension

Muscles tested : Hamstrings and quadriceps

Recommended Testing Protocol :

1) Speeds and repetitions (concentric)

   Athletes:

       a) 60°/s x 5 repetitions

       b) 240°/s to 300°/s x 25 repetitions

   Patients:

       a) 60°/s x 5 repetitions

       b) 180°/s x 25 repetitions

2) Rest between speeds : < 1 minute

3) First limbs tested : dominant or uninvolved

4) Rest between limbs : < 5 minutes

Joint : Ankle

Movement : Dorsiflexion and plantarflexion

Muscles tested : Dorsiflexors and plantarflexors

Recommended Testing Protocol :

    1) Speeds and repetitions (concentric)

   Athletes:

       a) 60°/s x 5 repetitions

       b) 180°/s x 25 repetitions

   Patients:

       a) 60°/s x 5 repetitions

       b) 180°/s x 25 repetitions

    2) Rest between speeds : < 1 minute

    3) First limbs tested : dominant or uninvolved

    4) Rest between limbs : < 5 minutes

Joint : Ankle

Movement : Inversion and eversion

Muscles tested : Ankle invertors and evertors

Recommended Testing Protocol :

    1) Speeds and repetitions (concentric)

       Athletes:

         a) 60°/s x 5 repetitions

         b) 180°/s x 25 repetitions

       Patients:

         a) 60°/s x 5 repetitions

         b) 180°/s x 25 repetitions

    2) Rest between speeds : < 1 minute

    3) First limbs tested : dominant or uninvolved

    4) Rest between limbs : < 5 minutes

Trunk

Movement : Trunk flexion and extension

Muscles tested : Trunk flexors and extensors

Recommended Testing Protocol :

    1) Speeds and repetitions (concentric)

       Athletes:

         a) 30°/s x 5 repetitions

         b) 120°/s x 25 repetitions

       Patients:

         a) 60°/s x 5 repetitions

         b) 120°/s x 25 repetitions

    2) Rest between speeds : < 1 minute

Joint : Shoulder

Movement : Flexion and extension

Muscles tested : Shoulder flexors and extensors

Recommended Testing Protocol :

    1) Speeds and repetitions (concentric)

      Athletes:

        a) 60°/s x 5 repetitions

        b) 240°/s x 25 repetitions

      Patients:

        a) 60°/s x 5 repetitions

        b) 180°/s x 25 repetitions

    2) Rest between speeds : < 1 minute

    3) First limbs tested : dominant or uninvolved

    4) Rest between limbs : < 5 minutes

Joint : Shoulder

Movement : Abduction and adduction

Muscles tested : Shoulder adductors and adductors

Recommended Testing Protocol :

    1) Speeds and repetitions (concentric)

      Athletes:

        a) 60°/s x 5 repetitions

        b) 240°/s x 25 repetitions

      Patients:

        a) 60°/s x 5 repetitions

        b) 180°/s x 25 repetitions

    2) Rest between speeds : < 1 minute

    3) First limbs tested : dominant or uninvolved

    4) Rest between limbs : < 5 minutes

Joint : Shoulder

Movement : Internal and external rotation

Muscles tested : Shoulder internal and external rotators (with 0° abduction)

Recommended Testing Protocol :

    1) Speeds and repetitions (concentric)

        Athletes:

          a) 60°/s x 5 repetitions

          b) 240°/s x 25 repetitions

        Patients:

          a) 60°/s x 5 repetitions

          b) 180°/s x 25 repetitions

    2) Rest between speeds : < 1 minute

    3) First limbs tested : dominant or uninvolved

    4) Rest between limbs : < 5 minutes

Joint : Shoulder

Movement : Horizontal abduction and adduction

Muscles tested : Shoulder horizontal abductors and adductors

Recommended Testing Protocol :

    1) Speeds and repetitions (concentric)

        Athletes:

          a) 60°/s x 5 repetitions

          b) 240°/s x 25 repetitions

        Patients:

          a) 60°/s x 5 repetitions

          b) 180°/s x 25 repetitions

    2) Rest between speeds : < 1 minute

    3) First limbs tested : dominant or uninvolved

    4) Rest between limbs : < 5 minutes

Joint : Elbow

Movement : Flexion and extension

Muscles tested : Elbow flexors and extensors

Recommended Testing Protocol :

    1) Speeds and repetitions (concentric)

        Athletes:

           a) 60°/s x 5 repetitions

           b) 240°/s x 25 repetitions

        Patients:

           a) 60°/s x 5 repetitions

           b) 180°/s x 25 repetitions

    2) Rest between speeds : < 1 minute

    3) First limbs tested : dominant or uninvolved

    4) Rest between limbs : < 5 minutes

Joint : Wrist

Movement : Flexion and extension

Muscles tested : Wrist flexors and extensors

Recommended Testing Protocol :

    1) Speeds and repetitions (concentric)

        Athletes:

           a) 60°/s x 5 repetitions

           b) 240°/s x 25 repetitions

        Patients:

           a) 60°/s x 5 repetitions

           b) 180°/s x 25 repetitions

    2) Rest between speeds : < 1 minute

    3) First limbs tested : dominant or uninvolved

    4) Rest between limbs : < 5 minutes

Joint : Wrist

Movement : Radial and ulnar deviations

Muscles tested : Wrist radial and ulnar deviators

Recommended Testing Protocol :

    1) Speeds and repetitions (concentric)

        Athletes:

          a) 60°/s x 5 repetitions

          b) 240°/s x 25 repetitions

        Patients:

          a) 60°/s x 5 repetitions

          b) 180°/s x 25 repetitions

    2) Rest between speeds : < 1 minute

    3) First limbs tested : dominant or uninvolved

    4) Rest between limbs : < 5 minutes

Joint : Hip

Movement : Flexion and extension

Muscles tested : Hip flexors and extensors

Recommended Testing Protocol :

    1) Speeds and repetitions (concentric)

        Athletes:

          a) 90°/s x 5 repetitions

          b) 180°/s x 25 repetitions

        Patients:

          a) 60°/s x 5 repetitions

          b) 180°/s x 25 repetitions

    2) Rest between speeds : < 1 minute

    3) First limbs tested : dominant or uninvolved

    4) Rest between limbs : < 5 minutes

Joint : Hip

Movement : Abduction and adduction

Muscles tested : Hip abductors and adductors

Recommended Testing Protocol :

1) Speeds and repetitions (concentric)

Athletes:

   a) 60°/s x 5 repetitions

   b) 180°/s x 25 repetitions

Patients:

   a) 60°/s x 5 repetitions

   b) 180°/s x 25 repetitions

2) Rest between speeds : < 1 minute

3) First limbs tested : dominant or uninvolved

4) Rest between limbs : < 5 minutes

A synopsis of training different muscle characteristics

Generally, athletes will complete a whole range of angular velocities within one training session. The intensity and duration of exercise need to be greater, with shorter rest periods than recommended for non-athletic patients.

Torque Training

Speed of training : low (60°/s)

Repetitions per set : few (5 repetitions)

Duration of exercise : long (20 to 30 minutes)

Range of movement : mid to full range

Force applied : maximum exertion

Work Training

Speed of training : fast (180°/s to 240°/s)

Repetitions per sets : many (25 to 50 repetitions)

Duration of exercise : long (20 to 25 minutes)

Range of movement : full range

Force applied : sustain the same intensity throughout the training session

Endurance training

Speed of training : fast ($180°/s$ to $240°/s$)

Repetitions per set : many (25 to 50 repetitions)

Duration of exercise : long (20 to 30 minutes)

Range of movement : mid to full range

Force applied : sustain the same intensity throughout the training session

Explosive power

Speed of training : any speed ($60°/s$ to $240°/s$)

Repetitions per sets : few (3 to 5 repetitions)

Duration of exercise : moderate (15 minutes)

Range of movement : initial range (first $10°$)

Force applied : maximum exertion, emphasis on explosiveness

G. Isokinetics and the testing of athletes

The following paragraphs will consider isokinetic testing of elite athletes in an attempt to clarify muscle strength characteristics of successful Asian athletes in a number of sports. The previous synopses gave background information on athletic profiling and talent identification in general. The present one focuses on local athletes. Most of the data have been collected during ongoing tests at the HKSI. Isokinetic training for athletes is recent at the HKSI. Data on the training of junior windsurfers and subsequent training responses, though limited, will be presented. Comments from the exercise physiologist and the conditioning coach will provide a subjective evaluation of the role of isokinetic strength training in the overall training program at the HKSI.

1. Isokinetic muscular profiles among Hong Kong elite male athletes

Aim: The purposes of this study were to investigate the isokinetic muscle characteristics of elite Hong Kong male athletes. The results from the different sports were then compared.

Subjects: Sixty-four male athletes participated in the study. Table 5-5 describes their personal characteristics and sports participation. Thirty males between the ages of 18 and 30, who had never taken part in regular training, served as controls. All subjects were painfree and injury free during the testing period. Subjects in the control group were included only if they had not sustained an injury within the prior 2 years.

Sport	Age (yrs)	Height (cm)	Weight (kg)
Badminton (n=11)	21.0 (3.3)	173.7(5.2)	63.6 (6.8)
Cycling (n=6)	23.0 (2.8)	172.0 (3.5)	63.0 (4.6)
Gymnastics (n=7)	18.0 (2.5)	167.4 (3.7)	59.6 (7.7)
Soccer (n=10)	26.7 (4.7)	173.0 (3.8)	67.0 (4.4)
Swimming (n=5)	18.8 (3.9)	177.4 (5.8)	72.0 (9.7)
Wheelchair athletes (n=4)	21.0 (4.0)	-	-
Controls (n=30)	21.0 (2.3)	167.9 (4.4)	59.1 (7.3)

Table 5-5 Personal characteristics (mean ± standard deviation).

Equipment: Cybex II+ with the UBXT and ankle plantar/dorsiflexion footplate were used.

Variables measured: Peak torque, total work, average power, peak torque acceleration energy, endurance ratio, agonist/antagonist ratio and work ratio were measured. Table 5-6 shows the movements measured for each of the sports. These were chosen because they reflected movements typical of the sports involved. Table 5-7 shows the test speeds and repetitions used for the tests. All tests were performed during the mid-season for each individual sport.

Test procedure: All three test movements were completed in one day, mainly because of limited availability of the elite athletes. Subjects were familiarized and stabilized. A test-specific warm-up proceeded the actual testing. A one-minute rest was given between the tests at the low and high speeds, and 3 minutes between contralateral testing. A 15-minute period was allowed between different joint movements. The non-dominant side was tested first.

Sport	Movement
Badminton	Knee extension and flexion
	Shoulder extension and flexion
Gymnastics	Knee extension and flexion
	Shoulder horizontal abduction and adduction
	Ankle plantarflexion and dorsiflexion
Soccer	Knee extension and flexion
	Ankle plantarflexion dorsiflexion
Swimming	Knee extension and flexion
	Shoulder extension and flexion
	Shoulder horizontal abduction and adduction
Cycling	Knee extension and flexion
	Ankle plantarflexion and dorsiflexion
Wheelchair	Shoulder extension and flexion
	Elbow extension and flexion

Table 5-6 Test movements used for each sport.

Movement	Low Speed ($°$/s)	Rep	Variable tested	High Speed ($°$/s)	Rep	Variable tested
Knee Extension/Flexion	60	5	Torque	180	50	Torque Work
Shoulder Extension/Flexion	60	5	Torque	240	25	Torque Work
Shoulder Horizontal Abduction/Adduction	60	5	Torque	240	25	Torque Work
Elbow Extension/Flexion	60	5	Torque	240	25	Torque Work
Ankle Plantarflexion/ Dorsiflexion	60	5	Torque	180	25	Torque Work

Table 5-7 The two test speeds used in each test movement.

Results: Selected data are shown in Table 5-8.

Sport	Movement	PT (Nm)	Agonist/ Anta-gonist Ratio (%)	Endurance Ratio (%)	PKTAE (J)
Badminton (n=11)	Knee extension	216 (34)	53 (7)	43 (8)	28 (5)
	Knee flexion	119 (22)		28 (13)	18 (8)
	Shoulder extension	98 (15)	69 (12)	59 (9)	27 (4)
	Shoulder flexion	64 (11)		70 (8)	22 (3)
Cycling (n=6)	Knee extension	231 (34)	51 (4)	63 (4)	27 (4)
	Knee flexion	117 (20)		41 (8)	13 (1)
	Ankle PF	112 (23)	30 (7)	43 (12)	11 (2)
	Ankle DF	29 (7)		35 (22)	4 (1)
Gymnastics (n=7)	Knee extension	184 (36)	40 (4)	60 (9)	36 (5)
	Knee flexion	91 (15)		53 (11)	17 (3)
	Shoulder horizontal abduction	68 (14)	85 (24)	76 (18)	20 (4)
	Shoulder horizontal adduction	73 (20)		75 (12)	27 (4)
	Ankle PF	84 (15)	48 (11)	55 (8)	9 (2)
	Ankle DF	30 (4)		55 (8)	5 (1)
Soccer (n=10)	Knee extension	184 (25)	60 (11)	41 (7)	23 (3)
	Knee flexion	113 (17)		35 (11)	14 (3)
	Ankle PF	100 (19)	36 (10)	53 (11)	10 (2)
	Ankle DF	31 (6)		44 (20)	5 (2)
Swimming (n=5)	Knee extension	211 (40)	54 (1)	71 (11)	42 (5)
	Knee flexion	113 (19)		46 (11)	24 (6)
	Shoulder extension	106 (22)	59 (6)	80 (9)	30 (7)
	Shoulder flexion	64 (12)		73 (12)	23 (6)
	Shoulder horizontal abduction	69 (17)	71 (9)	73 (12)	19 (5)
	Shoulder horizontal adduction	84 (20)		69 (12)	28 (8)
Wheelchair Racing (n=4)	Shoulder extension	90 (32)	69 (16)	64 (6)	25 (6)
	Shoulder flexion	72 (24)		57 (5)	22 (5)
	Elbow extension	52 (20)	121 (34)	73 (17)	13 (4)
	Elbow flexion	48 (14)		51 (17)	10 (3)

Control Group	Knee extension	170 (36)	56 (6)	41 (11)	22 (3)
(n=30)	Knee flexion	97 (21)		32 (15)	22 (3)
	Shoulder extension	67 (13)	76 (13)	47 (10)	18 (4)
	Shoulder flexion	48 (8)		55 (10)	16 (4)
	Shoulder horizontal adbuction	51 (9)	82 (15)	62 (10)	13 (3)
	Shoulder horizontal adduction	55 (13)		52 (12)	18 (4)
	Ankle PF	90 (19)	42 (11)	40 (10)	9 (2)
	Ankle DF	31 (6)		35 (13)	4 (1)
	Ebow extension	39 (12)	91 (15)	60 (12)	9 (2)
	Elbow flexion	39 (8)		59 (13)	10 (2)

Note: Ratios given are averages of individual ratios.
PT at 60°/s: 5 repetitions
Agonist/antagonist ratio, endurance ratio and PKTAE at 180°/s or 240°/s, see Table 5-7
Endurance ratio: 25 or 50 repetitions, see Table 5-7
PF: plantarflexion   DF: dorsiflexion

Table 5-8 Results of isokinetic testing of elite male Asian athletes (mean ± standard deviation).

a. Badminton (n=11)

Bilateral comparison of the knee flexors showed a significant difference in PT between the dominant and non-dominant sides when measured at high speed (Table 5-9). This was probably a consequence of habitual emphasis on one extremity during play. Badminton requires fast, frequent and powerful jumps and leaps. Knee extensor strength of badminton players was significantly greater than in other players. The shoulder extensors of badminton players demonstrated a significant bilateral difference in favor of the dominant side for all variables measured. Their shoulder flexors showed a significant bilateral difference for PT at 60°/s, and the same was true for TW and AP, but at the higher speed. The extension to flexion PT ratio was significantly greater on the non-dominant side, but most other variables measured were greater on the dominant side, as could be expected. Good shoulder extension strength, as measured in the players studied, is important for a fast and powerful game. Stewart (1977) indicated that the ability to generate force with the racquet, especially when reversing the direction of a fast moving ball, is highly dependent on the strength of the muscles involved. Shoulder flexion and extension strength is also crucial for a powerful execution of a serve and overhead action.

Groups	60°/s	180°/s
Control	58	45
Badminton	48	52
Cycling	45	38
Soccer	62	52

Table 5-9 Dominant side hamstrings/quadriceps peak torque ratio.

b. Cycling (n=6)

Bilateral comparison showed that the knee extensors of the dominant side generated significantly greater PT, TW and AP than the non-dominant side. This may lead to a cycling action which wastes energy, as differing levels of force are exerted on the pedals. The bicycle forward motion will be accelerating and decelerating in a cyclical way (LaFortune et al 1983). So (1991) suggested strengthening exercises for the weaker side, coupled with training for a more even technique. Cyclists generated high PT, PKTAE, TW and AP values for the knee extensors, confirming the role of this muscle group in generating a powerful pedal stroke. Obviously, as cycling requires a downward push and an upward pull, flexor muscle strength is also important. Hong Kong athletes demonstrated similar PT at 60°/s values for knee flexors as the control group, and therefore specific training of the cyclists' flexors was recommended. Cyclists had significantly stronger dominant side ankle dorsiflexors than plantarflexors at the slow speed test. This, again, may lower the efficiency of cycling. Their plantarflexors showed the highest PT, TW and AP at 180°/s. These muscles are needed for pushing the pedals continuously, and to oppose the ankle's tendency to flex upward as the foot exerts force on the pedal (Koch 1988).

c. Gymnastics (n=7)

Bilateral comparison showed a significant difference in knee extension PT, the non-dominant side being stronger at slow speed. This was expected, as gymnastics involves jumping and sprinting. They also had significantly greater PF torque on the non-dominant side, at fast speed, which again fits with the demands of the sport where the non-dominant foot is used for initiating a jump. Gymnasts scored high in ankle DF movement. A high value for dorsiflexion is desirable in this sport as ankle stability is important when jumping, landing and running. Bale and Goodway (1990) suggested that male gymnasts should pay great attention to strength and explosive power, particularly for the upper body.

d. Soccer (n=10)

Bilateral comparison showed no significant differences for the group as a whole, although the dominant leg of high standard players has been shown to be stronger (Kramer and Balsor 1990). All the muscle characteristics tested were similar to those obtained from the control group. Research has shown that high level players tend to have greater levels of strength in the lower limbs (Kramer and Balsor 1990).

e. Swimming (n=5)

Bilateral comparison showed no differences in PT for the knee extensors and flexors between the dominant and non-dominant sides, which were to be expected as both legs are needed to provide a balanced kick. The torques generated by the swimmers were similar to those of the other groups. Shoulder flexion was significantly greater on the dominant side. This may be caused by the breathing technique: swimmers turn their face to the dominant side while the shoulder is in flexion. As a result, the shoulder flexors of the dominant side work longer as the hand remains in the air. Shoulder horizontal abduction/adduction were greater in the swimmers' dominant side in nearly all variables tested, but significant differences were found only for horizontal adductor's PT and PKTAE, and horizontal abductor's TW, measured at 240°/s. Shoulder extension provides the majority of the propulsive force in all swimming strokes (Bloomfield 1986), and local studies have shown that there is a significant negative correlation between shoulder extension strength and swimming time (Chinese Sports Science Professionals National Research Institute of Sports Science 1988). The swimmers in this study had high shoulder extension PT values (measured at 60°/s and 240°/s), exceeding those measured in well trained Australian swimmers. The greater horizontal adduction strength found on the dominant side may have been also linked to the breathing style in swimming (So 1991). Shoulder abduction/adduction PT ratios for the slow and the fast speeds are presented in Table 5-8.

f. Wheelchair racing (n=4)

The PT ratios for the dominant shoulder extension/flexion for both sides in the slow speed torque test and non-dominant side in the fast speed torque test were significantly greater in wheelchair athletes than in the other athletes tested. This confirms the important role this muscle group plays in pushing the wheelchair. Shoulder flexion and extension has been found to be positively correlated to the wheelchair force generating capacity (Tupling and Davis 1983). Bilateral comparison of elbow extension and flexion resulted in no significant differences showing that more or less equal stress is exerted on the two arms, and that muscle strength, power and endurance will develop on both sides of the elbow with appropiate training.

For the group as a whole, with the exception of the gymnasts, gravity corrected H:Q ratio was within accepted limit. Note the influence of the test speed on subsequent results. Knee extension and flexion torques in male gymnasts, measured at a slow speed, were low and similar to the values attained by the control group. Gymnasts tend to stress the upper body more than the lower body. As gymnastics involves jumping and short sprinting, the flexors will be stressed more, leading to a lowered H:Q ratio. Athletes involved in running-based activities demonstrated, in general, greater knee flexor strength than athletes engaged in other sports. Running demands a strong hip extension, and, to produce this, the hamstrings need to be strong. Ankle PF and DF strength of Hong Kong elite athletes were not different from those of the control group, and values obtained were below those recorded in other countries. Again, the effect of the test speed is noticeable.

The results suggest that the torque values generated by the control group in the present study remained below those generated by youngsters from other ethnic backgrounds. Genetic makeup and lifestyle may be responsible for these differences. No significant bilateral differences were seen in shoulder extension and flexion for the athletic groups tested, whereas the control group showed significant bilateral differences for most of the variables measured. The dominant side was stronger. For all the groups and movements tested, only endurance ratio showed no statistically significant bilateral differences, while bilateral differences were found for all of the other variables measured. Further, these correlated well with muscle involvement in the particular sport, or general life activities (ie, in the control group). It is possible that the endurance ratio is a less sensitive measure of the effects of muscle training (So 1991).

The HKSI has been engaged in isokinetic testing of elite athletes for 8 years. Although more than 500 tests have been performed, given the structure and popularity of the various disciplines, many sports are under-represented. Tables 5-10 to 5-21 show data on sports where at least 7 athletes have been tested, together with sports for which there is very little isokinetic data available. The former includes tennis and badminton, and the latter canoeing, table-tennis, triathlon (women only) and the Chinese martial art Wu Shu. These data have been used to assess the relative weaknesses in muscle strength characteristics of individual sport participants. They have also been used as normative data for comparative purposes and in designing training programs to improve sports performance, as well as injury prevention.

TENNIS PLAYERS				
Dominant Side				
	Endurance (%)		**PKTAE (Joules)**	
	Extension	**Flexion**	**Extension**	**Flexion**
Males (n=9)	51.4	25.0	14.7	6.1
	(2.9)	(8.9)	(5.1)	(1.9)
Females (n=8)	50.0	26.9	14.8	6.3
	(10.7)	(22.0)	(3.1)	(2.9)

Table 5-10 Knee extension/flexion at 180°/s in tennis players (mean ± standard deviation).

TENNIS PLAYERS

Dominant Side

	Endurance (%)		PKTAE (Joules)	
	Abduction	**Adduction**	**Abduction**	**Adduction**
Males (n=9)	70.7	59.3	8.2	10.6
	(19.9)	(19.1)	(4.0)	(6.7)
Females (n=7)	63.0	73.4	8.0	10.3
	(21.1)	(14.2)	(2.5)	(3.2)

Table 5-11 Shoulder horizontal abduction/adduction at 240°/s in tennis players (mean ± standard deviation).

TRIATHLETES

Dominant Side

	Endurance (%)		PKTAE (Joules)	
	Extension	**Flexion**	**Extension**	**Flexion**
Females (n=4)	70.0	70.5	13.6	11.2
	(9.2)	(12.6)	(5.3)	(4.5)

Table 5-12 Shoulder extension/flexion at 240°/s in triathletes (mean ± standard deviation)

TABLE-TENNIS PLAYERS

Dominant Side

	Endurance (%)		PKTAE (Joules)	
	Internal	**External**	**Internal**	**External**
Males (n=4)	85.0	67.3	12.8	8.1
	(11.2)	(4.6)	(3.9)	(2.4)

Table 5-13 Shoulder internal/external rotation at 240°/s in table-tennis players (mean ± standard deviation).

TABLE-TENNIS PLAYERS

Dominant Side

	Endurance (%)		PKTAE (Joules)	
	Extension	Flexion	Extension	Flexion
Males (n=4)	47.0	29.0	23.8	11.3
	(2.9)	(9.0)	(2.7)	(2.2)

Table 5-14 Knee extension/flexion at 180°/s in table-tennis players (mean ± standard deviation).

TABLE-TENNIS PLAYERS

Dominant Side

	Endurance (%)		PKTAE (Joules)	
	Radial	Ulnar	Radial	Ulnar
Males (n=3)	58.0	57.7	1.8	1.4
	(14.7)	(18.8)	(0.6)	(0.3)

Table 5-15 Wrist radial/ulnar deviation at 180°/s in table-tennis players (mean ± standard deviation).

BADMINTON PLAYERS

Dominant Side

	Endurance (%)		PKTAE (Joules)	
	Extension	Flexion	Extension	Flexion
Males (n=11)	59.3	70.1	26.7	22.2
	(8.9)	(8.1)	(3.5)	(3.2)
Females (n=7)	60.7	70.4	13.2	12.5
	(9.9)	(9.0)	(3.5)	(2.9)

Table 5-16 Shoulder extension/flexion at 240°/s in badminton players (mean ± standard deviation).

BADMINTON PLAYERS

Dominant Side

	Endurance (%)		PKTAE (Joules)	
	Extension	**Flexion**	**Extension**	**Flexion**
Males (n=11)	76.6	62.1	2.3	3.1
	(12.7)	(9.3)	(0.6)	(0.6)
Females (n=7)	52.3	70.8	13.2	12.5
	(32.0)	(8.7)	(3.5)	(2.9)

Table 5-17 Wrist extension/flexion at 180°/s in badminton players (mean ± standard deviation).

CANOEIST

Dominant Side

	Endurance (%)		Total Work (Joules)		PKTAE (Joules)	
	Extension	**Flexion**	**Extension**	**Flexion**	**Extension**	**Flexion**
Males (n=5)	80.4	77.2	2949.2	1669.0	44.1	27.0
	(6.2)	(5.0)	(434.8)	(273.5)	(9.9)	(5.2)

Table 5-18 Shoulder extension/flexion at 240°/s in canoeist (mean ± standard deviation).

CANOEIST

Dominant Side

	Endurance (%)		Total Work (Joules)		PKTAE (Joules)	
	Extension	**Flexion**	**Extension**	**Flexion**	**Extension**	**Flexion**
Males (n=5)	91.0	86.0	1437.2	1024.6	15.0	13.1
	(13.1)	(9.7)	(373.9)	(217.4)	(2.0)	(3.5)

Table 5-19 Elbow extension/flexion at 180°/s in canoeists (mean ± standard deviation).

WU SHU PLAYERS

Dominant Side

| | Endurance (%) | | PKTAE (Joules) | |
	Plantarflexion	Dorsiflexion	Plantarflexion	Dorsiflexion
Males (n=4)	39.0	35.5	9.9	3.7
	(10.7)	(28.2)	(0.7)	(0.7)
Females (n=4)	34.3	40.7	6.7	3.0
	(3.0)	(2.9)	(1.8)	(0.5)

Table 5-20 Ankle plantarflexion/dorsiflexion at 180°/s in Wu Shu players (mean ± standard deviation).

WU SHU PLAYERS

Dominant Side

| | Endurance (%) | | PKTAE (Joules) | |
	Extension	Flexion	Extension	Flexion
Females (n=4)	54.0	47.7 1	4.6	9.3
	(20.8)	(37.2)	(2.9)	(3.6)

Table 5-21 Knee extension/flexion at 180°/s in Wu Shu players (mean ± standard deviation).

Table 5-22 illustrates movements performed by athletes from different sports. The movements chosen were regarded as specific to the movement patterns and strength requirements in each sport. Variables measured included peak torque, peak % body weight ratio, work, total work, average work, power, average power, peak torque acceleration energy, and endurance ratio.

Movement	Sport
Shoulder horizontal abduction/adduction	Tennis, Swimming, Soccer
Shoulder internal/external rotation	Triathlon, Swimming, Table-tennis
Shoulder flexion/extension	Triathlon, Badminton, Bowling, Canoeing
Elbow flexion/extension	Canoeing
Wrist flexion/extension	Badminton
Wrist radial/ulnar deviation	Tennis
Back flexion/extension	Triathlon, Badminton, Bowling, Canoeing
Hip flexion/extension	Triathlon
Knee flexion/extension	Triathlon, Swimming, Table-tennis, Tennis, Badminton, Bowling, Wu Shu, Soccer
Ankle plantar/dorsiflexion	Triathlon, Wu Shu, Soccer

Table 5-22 A synopsis of the movements in sport performed at HKSI.

2. Construction of an isokinetic training program for athletes

The scientific literature regarding the construction of an isokinetic training program for sport-related strength training is scarce. Information on how to decide which speeds, repetitions, sets and rest periods to use is not available. At the HKSI, isokinetic training practices are jointly based on the rehabilitation model, and on the general principles which govern athletic training. Isokinetic training at the HKSI involves velocity spectrum training, which, for example for the rowers, is based on initial tests on a rowing ergometer to establish actual rowing-specific speeds of movement. Initial isokinetic tests provide guidance in the construction of a training program, including movements, speeds and muscle characteristics to be emphasized. At the same time any bilateral differences can be rectified. Isolated experiments at the HKSI with individual athletes, for example one rower, have suggested that optimal training results may be gained by adding isokinetic training into the existing strength training program once per week, resulting in four weekly strength training sessions (So 1995, personal communications). Strength training for more than four times per week may lead to overtraining. These findings are purely anecdotal, and not the result of objective evaluation. It is typical for rowers and windsurfers to train with weights three times per week. The HKSI is presently using isokinetics to supplement the strength training program of a group of junior windsurfers and soccer players. Tables 5-23 to 5-25 describe their isokinetic strength training programs.

Speed(°/s)	Repetitions per set	Rest(sec) between sets
60	4	30
60	4	50
90	5	30
120	10	55
180	20	50
60	4	-

Table 5-23 Elbow extension/flexion program for junior windsurfers.

Speed (°/s)	Repetitions per set	Rest (sec) between sets
60	5	40
60	5	40
120	10	90
180	20	90
90	5	120
60	5	40
60	5	40
120	10	40
180	20	120
60	5	

Table 5-24 Trunk flexion/extension program for junior windsurfers.

Speed(°/s)	Repetitions per set	Rest between sets (sec)
60	4	30

Table 5-25 Knee flexion/extension training program (6 weeks) of elite junior soccer player.

Information of the physiological responses of the athletes to the training bout are measured using variables, such as blood lactate and creatine kinase. In the short-term, they allow adjustments to be made to the training regime, especially in terms of intensity. Such tests should also allow intra and inter-individual comparisons to be made over a period of time regarding training induced improvements.

3. Training related changes in isokinetic strength: some preliminary data

The effectiveness of concentric and eccentric isokinetic knee extension/flexion training was studied at the HKSI to determine whether this could improve functional performance, assessed by vertical jump, standing long-jump and 50-meter sprint performance, and the stability of the knee in 14 elite junior soccer players. The players were divided into the concentric (Con) and eccentric (Ecc) training groups, and trained twice per week for 6 weeks. The training protocol employed is shown in Table 5-25. After the 6-week training period, both groups were re-tested. Besides the functional tests, one set of four maximal effort repetitions of concentric knee extension/flexion movements were completed at $30°/s, 60°/s, 90°/s, 120°/s, 180°/s$ and $240°/s$. Data analysis showed some significant strength gains as measured by peak torque, H:Q ratio, TW, H:Q ratio in PT, peak torque body weight ratio (PT % BW) and total work/body weight ratio (TW % BW) following both concentric and eccentric training regime. Statistically significant improvements were found for VJ in the Con group but not for the Ecc group.

The exercise physiologist and the conditioning coach at the HKSI would advocate the use of isokinetic training as a supplementary strength training exercise, though little data exist to substantiate this view. At this stage, they would not recommend athletes to replace isoinertial resistance training completely with isokinetic training (So and Tse, personal communications, 1995). In many cases, isokinetic machines are not widely available, and a further limitation is the need for qualified personnel in assisting with all phases of a bout of training. It also takes a considerable amount of time to train different body parts within one session. For example, training one motion of the upper limbs will easily take 30 minutes. Further, the planes of possible movement are more limited with isokinetic machines than with free weights. Eccentric training has not been used at the HKSI yet. This is mainly because such specific training is seen as unnatural in many sports, and coaches are reluctant to let their athletes undertake training of which the effects are largely unknown. A study on isokinetic eccentric training is now under way. Sports such as powerlifting is generally considered as one which potentially may benefit from specific eccentric training. The opinion of the resident conditioning coach at the HKSI is that isokinetic training can mimic the actual speeds and joint angles inherent in particular sports, making isokinetics potentially very sport-specific. Isokinetics may have an important place in the strength training in weight category sports, and sports in which the body weight has to be carried or "lifted", as isokinetic strength gains appear not to induce muscle hypertrophy, but neural adaptations instead (Tse 1995, personal communications). However, little scientific evidence exists, and further, more detailed and well controlled studies are planned.

References

1. Abe T, Kawakami Y, Ikegawa S, et al. Isometric and isokinetic knee joint performance in Japanese alpine ski racers. J Sports Med Phys Fitness 32: 353-357, 1992.

2. Abernethy P, Wilson G, Logan P. Strength and power assessment: Issues, controversies and challenges. Sports Med 19(6): 401-417, 1995.

3. Addison R, Schultz A. Trunk strengths in patients seeking hospitalization for chronic low back disorders. Spine 5(6): 539-544, 1980.

4. Albert M. Physiologic and clinical principles of eccentrics. In Albert M (Ed) Eccentric Muscle Training in Sports and Orthopedics. 2nd edition, 23-35, 1995.Churchill Livingstone, London.

5. Alderink GJ, Kuck DJ. Isokinetic shoulder strength of high school and college-aged pitchers. J Orthop Sports Phys Ther 7: 163-172, 1986.

6. Alexander MJ. The relationship between muscle strength and sprint kinematics in elite sprinters. Can J Sport Sci 14: 148-157, 1989.

7. Anderson MA, Gieck JH, Perrin D, et al. The relationship among isometric, isotonic, and isokinetic concentric and eccentric quadriceps and hamstring force and three components of athletic performance. J Orthop Sports Phys Ther 14(3): 114-120, 1991.

8. Astrand P, Rodahl K. Textbook of Work Physiology: Physiological Bases of Exercise. 3rd edition, 1986. McGraw-Hill International Editions, New York.

9. Bale P, Goodway J. Performance variables associated with the competitive gymnast. Sports Med 10(3): 139-145, 1990.

10. Baltzopoulos V, Brodie DA. Isokinetic dynamometry: Applications and limitations. Sports Med 8(2): 101-116, 1989.

11. Bandy WD, McLaughlin S. Intramachine and intermachine reliability for selected dynamic muscle performance tests. J Orthop Sports Phys Ther 18: 609-613, 1993.

12. Behm DG, Sale DG. Intended rather than actual movement velocity determines velocity-specific training response. J Appl Physiol 74: 359-368, 1993.

13. Bell GJ, Snydmiller GD, Neary JP, et al. The effect of high and low velocity resistance training on anaerobic power output in cyclists. J Human Movement Studies 16: 173-181, 1989.

14. Bemben MG, Grump KJ, Massey BH. Assessment of technical accuracy of the Cybex II isokinetic dynamometer and analog recording system. J Orthop Sports Phys Ther 7(4): 12-17, 1988.

15. Bennett JG, Stauber WT. Evaluation and treatment of anterior knee pain using eccentric exercise. Med Sci Sports Exerc 18(5): 526-530, 1986.

16. Berg K, Blanke D, Miller M. Muscular fitness profile of female college basketball players. J Orthop Sports Phys Ther 7: 59-64, 1985.

17. Bloomfield J, Blansky BA, Acland TR, et al. The mechanical and physiological characteristics of pre-adolescent swimmers, tennis players and non-competitors. In Day JAP (Ed) Human Kinetics 165-176, 1986. Illinois, Champaign.

18. Bohannon RW. Hand-held compared with isokinetic dynamometry for measurement of static knee extension torque (parallel reliability of dynamometers). Clin Phys Physiol Meas 11:(3) 217-222, 1990.

19. Broccoletti P. Building, 1981. Icarus Press, South Bend, Indiana.

20. Burdett RG, VanSwearingen J. Reliability of isokinetic muscle endurance tests. J Orthop Sports Phys Ther 8: 484-488, 1987.

21. Burnett CN, Betts EF, King WM. Reliability of isokinetic measurements of hip muscle torque in young boys. Phys Ther 70:244-249, 1990

22. Burnham RS, Gordon B, Olenik L, et al. Shoulder abduction strength measurment in football players: Reliability and validity of two field tests. Clin J Sports Med 5:90-94, 1995.

23. Burnie J, Brodie DA. Isokinetics in the assessment of rehabilitation. Clin Biomech 1: 140-146, 1986.

24. Bynum EB, Barrack RL, Alexander AH. Open versus closed chain kinetic exercises after anterior cruciate ligament reconstruction: A prospective randomized study. Am J Sports Med 23(4): 401-406, 1995.

25. Cabri JMH. Isokinetic strength aspects of human joints and muscles. Critical Reviews in Biomedical Engineering 19(2,3): 231-259, 1991.

26. Cahill BR, Griffith EH. Effect of preseason conditioning on the incidence and severity of high school football knee injuries. Am J Sports Med 6: 180-184, 1978.

27. Caiozzo VJ, Perrine JJ, Edgerton VR. Training-induced alteration of the in vivo force-velocity relationship of human muscle. J Appl Physiol 51: 750-754, 1981.

28. Campbell DE, Wayne G. Foot-pounds of torque of the normal knee and the rehabilitated postmeniscectomy knee. Phys Ther 59: 418-421, 1979.

29. Carlsoo S, Fohlin L, Skoglund G. Studies of co-contraction of knee muscles. In Desmedt JE (Ed) New developments in electromyography and clin neurophysiology 648-655, Karger, Basel, 1973.

30. Cawthorn M, Cummings G, Walker JR, et al. Isokinetic measurement of foot invertor and evertor force in three positions of plantarflexion and dorsiflexion. J Orthop Sports Phys Ther 14: 75-81, 1991.

31. Cetti R. Conservative treatment of injury to the fibular ligament of the ankle. Br J Sports Med 16(1): 52-67, 1982

32. Chick RR, Jackson DW. Tears of the anterior cruciate ligament in young athletes. J Bone Joint Surg 10: 970-973, 1978.

33. Costill DL, Coyle EF, Fink WF, et al. Adaptation in skeletal muscle following strength training. J Appl Physiol 46: 96-99, 1979.

34. Costill DL, Daniels J, Evans W, et al. Skeletal muscle enzymes and fiber composition in male and female track athletes. J Appl Physiol 40: 149-154, 1976.

35. Costill DL, Fink WJ, Habansky AJ. Muscle rehabilitation following knee surgery. Physician Sports Med 5: 71-74, 1977.

36. Cote C, Simoneau JA, Lagasse P, et al. Isokinetic strength training protocols: Do they induce skeletal muscle fiber hypertrophy? Arch Phys Med Rehabil 69: 281-285, 1988.

37. Coyle EF, Feiring DC, Rotkins TC, et al. Specificity of power improvements through slow and fast isokinetic training. J Appl Physiol 51: 1437-1442, 1981.

38. D'Orazio B (Ed). Back Pain Rehabilitation, 1993. Andover Medical Publishers, USA.

39. Davies AH. Chronic effects of isokinetic and allokinetic training on muscle force, endurance, and muscular hypertrophy. Temple University (Philadelphia) Physical Education Department Doctoral Dissertation. Diss Abs Int 38: 153A, 1977.

40. Davies CT, Thompson MW. Physiological responses to prolonged exercise in ultramarathon athletes. J Appl Physiol 61(2): 611-617, 1986.

41. Davies GJ. A Compendium of Isokinetics in Clinical Usage and Rehabilitation Techniques. 2nd edition, 1984. S & S Publisher, La Crosse, USA.

42. Dean E. Physiology and therapeutic implications of negative work. Phys Ther 68: 233-237, 1988.

43. DeCarlo MS, Shelbourne KD, McCarroll JR, et al. Traditional versus accelerated rehabilitation following ACL reconstruction: A one-year follow-up. J Orthop Sports Phys Ther 15(6): 309-316, 1992.

44. DeLee JC, Drez D. Orthopedic Sports Medicine: Principles and Practice. Vol 1 & 2, 1994. WB Saunders Comp., USA.

45. Delitto A, Rose SJ, Crandell CE, et al. Reliability of isokinetic measurements of trunk muscle performance. Spine 16(7): 800-803, 1991.

46. Diamond JE. Rehabilitation of ankle sprains. Clin Sports Med 8(4): 877-889, 1989.

47. Drez D, Paine R, Neuschwander DC. In vivo testing of closed versus open kinetic chain exercises in patients with documented tears of the anterior cruciate ligament. Orthop Trans 16: 43, 1992.

48. Duncan PW, Chandler JM, Cavanaugh DK, et al. Mode and speed specificity of eccentric and concentric exercise training. J Orthop Sports Phys Ther 11(2): 70-75, 1989.

49. Durand A, Malouin F, Richards CL, et al. Intertrial reliability of work measurements recorded during concentric isokinetic knee extension and flexion in subjects with and without meniscal tears. Phys Ther 71(11): 804-812, 1991.

50. Dvir Z. Isokinetics: Muscle testing, interpretation and clinical applications, 1995. Churchill Livingstone, London.

51. Eckhardt R, Scharf HP, Puhl W. Metabolic and hemodynamic investigations during isokinetic and ergometric load programs, measured in 21 healthy subjects [Abs]. Int J Sports Med 12: 112, 1991.

52. Ellenbecker TS, Davies GJ, Rowinske MJ. Concentric versus eccentric isokinetic strengthening of the rotator cuff: Objective data versus functional test. Am J Sports Med 16(1): 64-69, 1988.

53. Elliot J. Assessing muscle strength isokinetically. J Am Med Assoc 240: 2408-2410, 1978.

54. Enoka RM. Muscle strength and its development: New perspectives. Sports Med 6: 146-168, 1988.

55. Eriksson E. Rehabilitation of muscle function after sports injury: Major problem in Sports Medicine. Int J Sports Med 2: 1-6, 1981.

56. Eriksson E, Haggmark T. A comparison of isometric muscle training and electrical stimulation in the recovery after knee ligament surgery. Am J Sports Med 7: 169-171, 1979.

57. Esselman PC, DeLateur BJ, Alquist AD, et al. Torque development in isokinetic training. Arch Phys Med Rehabil 72: 723-728, 1991.

58. Ewing JL, Wolfe DR, Rogers MA, et al. Effects of velocity of isokinetic training on strength, power, and quadriceps muscle fiber characteristics. Eur J Appl Physiol 61: 159-162, 1990.

59. Farrell M, Richards JG. Analysis of the reliability and validity of the kinetic communicator exercise device. Med Sci Sports Exerc 18(1): 44-49, 1986.

60. Feiring DC, Ellenbecker TS, Derscheid GL. Test-re-test reliability of the Biodex isokinetic dynamometer. J Orthop Sports Phys Ther 11(7): 298-300, 1990.

61. Figoni SF, Christ CB, Massey BH. Effects of speed, hip and knee angle, and gravity on hamstring to quadriceps torque ratios. J Orthop Sports Phys Ther 9(8): 287-291, 1988.

62. Fridén J, Seger J, Sjöström M, et al. Adaptive response in human skeletal muscle subjected to prolonged eccentric training. Int J Sports Med 4: 177-183, 1983.

63. Friedlander AL, Genant HK, Sadowski S, et al. A 2-year program of aerobics and weight training enhances bone mineral density of young women. J Bone Miner Res 10: 574-585, 1995.

64. Frisiello S, Gazaille A, O'Halloran J, et al. Test-re-test reliability of eccentric peak torque values for shoulder medial and lateral rotation using the Biodex isokinetic dynamometer. J Orthop Sports Phys Ther 19(6): 341-344, 1994.

65. Frontera WR, Hughes VA, Dallal GE, et al. Reliability test in 45- to 78-year-old men and women. Arch Phys Med Rehabil 74: 1181-1185, 1993.

66. Fry AC, Kraemer WJ, Weseman CA, et al. Effects of an off-season strength and conditioning program on starters and non-starters in women's collegiate volleyball. J Appl Sport Sci Res 5: 174-181, 1991.

67. Frymoer JW, Pope MH, Clements JH, et al. Risk factors in low back pain. J Bone Joint Surg 65A(2): 213-217, 1983.

68. Garn SN, Newton RA. Kinesthetic awareness in subjects with multiple ankle sprains. Phys Ther 68(11): 1667-1671, 1988.

69. Garnica RA. Muscular power in young women after slow and fast isokinetic training. J Orthop Sports Phys Ther 8: 1-9, 1986.

70. Garrett WE, Mumma M, Lucareche CL. Ultrastructural differences in human skeletal muscle fiber types. Orthop Clin North Am 14: 413-425, 1983.

71. Gettman LR, Carter LA, Strathman TA. Physiologic changes after 20 weeks of isotonic versus isokinetic circuit training. J Sports Med 20: 265-275, 1980.

72. Gilliam T, Sady S, Freeson P, et al. Isokinetic torque level for high school football players. Arch Phys Med Rehabil 60: 110-114, 1979.

73. Giove TP, Miller SJ, Kent BE, et al. Non-operative treatment of torn anterior cruciate ligament. J Bone Joint Surg 65A: 184-192, 1983.

74. Gleeson NP, Mercer TH. Reproducibility of isokinetic leg strength and endurance characteristics of adult men and women. Eur J Appl Phys 65: 221-228, 1992.

75. Gleim G, Nicholas J, Webb J. Isokinetic evaluation following leg injuries. Physician Sports Med 6: 75-82, 1978.

76. Golden C, Dudley G. Strength after bouts of eccentric or concentric actions. Med Sci Sports Exerc 24: 926-933, 1992.

77. Grabiner MD, Jeziorowski JJ, Divekar AD. Isokinetic measurements of trunk extension and flexion performance collected with the Biodex clinical data station. J Orthop Sports Phys Ther 11: 590-598, 1990.

78. Grace DL. Lateral ankle ligament injuries. Clin Orthop Related Res 183: 153-159, 1984.

79. Grace TG, Sweetser ER, Nelson MA, et al. Isokinetic muscle imbalance and knee-joint injuries. J Bone Joint Surg 66A(5): 734-739, 1984.

80. Gransberg L, Knuttson E. Determination of dynamic muscle strength in man with acceleration controlled isokinetic movements. Acta Phys Scand 119: 317-320, 1983.

81. Gray JW, Chandler JM. Percent decline in peak torque production during repeated concentric and eccentric contractions of the quadriceps femoris muscle. J Orthop Sports Phys Ther 11: 309-314, 1989.

82. Greenfield BH, Donatelli R, Wooden MJ, et al. Isokinetic evaluation of shoulder rotational strength between the plane of scapula and the frontal plane. Am J Sports Med 18: 124-128, 1990.

83. Griffin JW. Differences in elbow flexion torque measured concentrically, eccentrically, and isometrically. Phys Ther 67: 1205-1208, 1987.

84. Grimby G. Clinical aspects of strength and power training. In Komi PV (Ed) Strength and Power in Sport 338-354, 1992. Blackwell Scientific Publications, London.

85. Grimby G. Progressive resistance exercise for injury rehabilitation: Special emphasis on isokinetic training. Sports Med 2: 309-315, 1985.

86. Grimby G, Gustafsson E, Peterson K, et al. Quadriceps function and training after knee ligament surgery. Med Sci Sports Exerc 12: 70-75, 1980.

87. Gydikov A. Patterns of discharge of different types of alpha motor neurons and motor units during voluntary and reflex activities under normal physiological conditions. In Komi PV (Ed) Biomechanics VAB, 1976. University Park Press, Baltimore.

88. Häkkinen K, Komi PV, Kauhanen K. Electromyographic and force production characteristics of leg extension muscles of elite weightlifters during isometric, concentric, and various stretch-shortening cycle exercises. Int J Sports Med 7: 144-151, 1986.

89. Hamilton WG, Hamilton LH, Marshall P, et al. A profile of the musculoskeletal characteristics of elite professional ballet dancers. Am J Sport Med 20(3): 267-273, 1992.

90. Harding B, Black T, Bruulsema A, et al. Reliability of a reciprocal test protocol performed on the Kinetic Communicator: An isokinetic test of knee extensor and flexor strength. J Orthop Sports Phys Ther 10: 218-223, 1988.

91. Harman E. The biomechanics of resistance exercise. In Baechle TR (Ed) Essentials of strength training and conditioning 19-50, 1994. National Strength and Conditioning Association. Human Kinetics Publishers, Champaign.

92. Hause M, Fujiwara M, Kikuchi S. A new method of quantitative measurement of abdominal and back muscle strength. Spine 5(2): 143-148, 1980.

93. Heitman RJ, Kovaleski JE. Test-rest reliability of isokinetic knee extension and flexion torque measurements in persons who are mentally retarded. Clin Kinesiology 47: 17-20, 1993.

94. Henning CE, Lych MA, Glick JR. An in vivo strain gauge study of elongation of the anterior cruciate ligament. Am J Sports Med 13(1): 22-26, 1985.

95. Higbie EJ, Cureton KJ, Warren GL. Effects of concentric and eccentric training on muscle strength, cross-sectional area and neural activation [Abs]. Med Sci Sports Exerc 26(5) (Suppl): S31, 1994.

96. Hinton RY. Isokinetic evaluation of shoulder rotational strength in high school baseball pitchers. Am J Sports Med 16: 274-279, 1988.

97. Hislop HJ, Perrine JJ. The isokinetic concept of exercise. Phys Ther 47: 114-117, 1967.

98. Horstmann T, Mayer F, Fischer J, et al. The cardiocirculatory reaction to isokinetic exercises in dependence on the form of exercise and age. Int J Sports Med 15: S50-S55, 1994.

99. Huijing PA. Mechanical muscle models. In Komi PV (Ed) Strength and Power in Sport 130-150, 1992. Blackwell Scientific Publications, London.

100. Hurley JM, Hagberg JM, Holloszy BF. Muscle weakness among elite powerlifters. Med Sci Sports Exerc (Suppl) 20: S81, 1988.

101. Ikai M, Fukunaga T. A study of training effect on strength per unit cross-sectional area of muscle by means of ultrasonic measurement. Int Z Angew Physiol 28: 172, 1970.

102. Jablonowsky R, Inbar O, Rotstein A, et al. Evaluation of anaerobic performance capacity by the isokinetic Ariel computerized exercise system: Reliability and validity. J Sports Med Phys Fitness 32(3): 262-270, 1992.

103. Jensen K, Fabio RPD. Evaluation of eccentric exercise in treatment of patellar tendinitis. Phys Ther 69(3): 211-216, 1989.

104. Jensen RC, Warren B, Laursen C, et al. Static pre-load effect on knee extensor isokinetic concentric and eccentric performance. Med Sci Sports Exerc 23(1): 10-14, 1991.

105. Jobe FW, Tibone JE, Perry J, et al. An EMG analysis of the shoulder in throwing and pitching: A preliminary report. Am J Sports Med 11: 3, 1983.

106. Johnson D. Controlling anterior shear during isokinetic knee extension exercise. J Orthop Sports Phys Ther 4: 23-31, 1982.

107. Johnson J, Siegel D. Reliability of an isokinetic movement of the knee extensors. Res Q 49(1): 88-90, 1978.

108. Jones DA, Rutherford OM. Human muscle strength training: The effects of three different training regimes and the nature of the resultant changes. J Physiol 391: 1-11, 1987.

109. Jonhagen S, Nemeth G, Eriksson E. Hamstring injuries in sprinters: The role of concentric and eccentric hamstring muscle strength and flexibility. Am J Sports Med 22(2): 262-266, 1994.

110. Kanehisa H, Miyashita M. Specificity of velocity in strength training. Eur J Appl Physiol 5: 104-106, 1983.

111. Kannus P. Isokinetic evaluation of muscular performance: Implications for muscle testing and rehabilitation. Int J Sports Med 15: S11-S18, 1994.

112. Kannus P. Types of injury prevention. In Renström PAFH (Ed) Sports Injuries: Basic Principles of Prevention and Care 16-23, 1993. Blackwell Scientific Publications, London.

113. Kannus P. Relationship between peak torque, peak angular impulse, and average power in thigh muscle of subjects with knee damage. Res Q Exerc Sports 61: 141-145, 1990.

114. Kannus P. Ratio of hamstring to quadriceps femoris muscles' strength in the anterior cruciate ligament. Phys Ther 68(6): 961-965, 1988.

115. Kannus P, Järvinen M. Knee flexor/extensor strength ratio in follow-up of acute knee distortion injuries. Arch Phys Med Rehabil 71: 38-41, 1990.

116. Kannus P, Järvinen M. Prediction of torque, peak torque acceleration energy and power of thigh muscle from peak torque. Med Sci Sports Exerc 21: 304-307, 1989.

117. Kannus P, Kaplan M. Angle-specific torques of thigh muscles: Variability analysis in 200 healthy adults. Can J Sports Sci 16: 264-270, 1991.

118. Karnofel H, Wilkinson K, Lentell G. Reliability of isokinetic muscle testing at the ankle. J Orthop Sports Phys Ther 11:150-154, 1989.

119. Kaufman KR, An KN, Litchy WJ, et al. Dynamic joint forces during knee isokinetic exercise. Am J Sports Med 19: 305-316, 1991.

120. Kaumeyer G, Malone T. Ankle injuries: Anatomical and biomechanical considerations necessary for the development of an injury prevention program. J Orthop Sports Phys Ther 1(3): 171-177, 1980.

121. Kawakami Y, Kanehisa H, Ikegqwa S, et al. Concentric and eccentric strength during and after fatigue in 13 year-old boys. Eur J Appl Physiol 67: 121-124, 1993.

122. Kellis E, Baltzopoulos V. Isokinetic eccentric exercise. Sports Med 19(3): 202-222, 1995.

123. Kilfoil MR, St. Pierre. Reliability of Cybex II isokinetic evaluations of torque in post-poliomyelitis syndrome. Arch Phys Med Rehabil 74:730-735, 1993.

124. Klausen K. The form and function of the loaded human spine. Acta Physiol Scand 65: 176-190, 1965.

125. Klissouras V. Heritability of adaptive variation. J Appl Physiol 31: 338, 1971.

126. Klopfer DA, Greij SD. Examining quadriceps/hamstrings performance at high velocity isokinetics in untrained subjects. J Orthop Sports Phys Ther 10: 18-22, 1988.

127. Knapik JJ, Bauman CL, Jones BH, et al. Preseason strength and flexibility imbalances associated with athletic injuries in female collegiate athletes. Am J Sports Med 19(1): 76-80, 1991.

128. Knight KL (Ed). Strength imbalance and knee injury. Phys Sports Med 8: 140, 1980.

129. Koch C. Power, strength and endurance are only part of the story: The real key to cycling is efficiency. Bicycle Guide March, 36-49, 1988.

130. Komadel L. The identification of performance potential. In Dirix A, Knuttgen HG, Tittel K (Eds) The Olympic Book of Sports Medicine 275-285, 1988. Blackwell Scientific Publications, London.

131. Komi PV. Physiological and biomechanical correlates of muscle function: Effects of muscle structure and stretch-shortening cycle on force and speed. Exerc Sports Sci Rev 81, 1984. Terijung, RL Ed, Lexington.

132. Komi PV, Suominen H, Heikkinen E, et al. Effects of heavy resistance training and explosive type strength training methods on mechanical, functional and metabolic aspects of performance. In Komi VP (Ed) Exercise and Sports Biology, 90-102, 1982. Human Kinetics, Champaign.

133. Komi PV, Viitasalo JT. Changes in motor unit activity and metabolism in human skeletal muscle during and after repeated eccentric and concentric contractions. Acta Physiol Scand 100: 246-254, 1977.

134. Koplan JP, Siscovick DS, Goldbaum GM. The risk of exercise: A public health view of injuries and hazards. Public Health Rep 100: 189-195, 1985.

135. Korkia P, Tunstall PD, Maffulli N. Epidemiologic study of training related injuries in triathletes. Br J Sports Med 28(3): 191-196, 1994.

136. Kramer JF. Reliability of knee extensor and flexion torques during continuous concentric-eccentric cycles. Arch Phys Med Rehabil 71: 460-464, 1990.

137. Kramer JF, Balsor BE. Lower extremity preference and knee extensor torques in intercollegiate soccer players. Can J Sport Sci 15(3): 180-184, 1990.

138. Kramer JF, Nusca D, Fowler P, et al. Knee flexor and extensor strength during concentric and eccentric muscle actions after anterior cruciate ligament reconstruction using the semitendinosus tendon and ligament augmentation device. Am J Sports Med 21(2): 285-291, 1993.

139. Krazier KL, Holbrook TL, Kelsey JL, et al. The frequency of occurrence, impact, and cost of musculoskeletal conditions in the United States. Am Academy Orthop Surgeons,Chicago, 1984.

140. Kues JM, Rothstein JM, Lamb RL. Obtaining reliable measurements of knee extensior torque produced during maximal voluntary contractions: An experimental investigation. Phys Ther 72(7):492-504, 1992.

141. La-Fortune MA, Cavanagh PP, Villiant GA, et al. A study of the riding mechanics of elite cyclists. Med Sci Sports Exerc 15: 113, 1983.

142. Lagasse PP, Katch FI, Katch VL, et al. Reliability and validity of the Omnitron Hydraulic Resistance Exercise and Testing Device. Int J Sports Med 10(6): 445-458, 1989.

143. Laird CE, Rozier CK. Toward understanding the terminology of exercise mechanics. Phys Ther 59: 287-292, 1979.

144. Larson CB. Pathomechanics of backache. J Iowa Med Soc 51: 643-650, 1961.

145. Leroux JL, Codine P, Thomas E, et al. Isokinetic evaluation of rotational strength in normal shoulders and shoulders with impingement syndrome. Clin Orthop Related Res 304: 108-115, 1994.

146 Lesmes GR, Costill DL, Coyle EF, et al. Muscle strength and power changes during maximal isokinetic training. Med Sci Sports 10: 266-269, 1978.

147. Levene JA, Hart BA, Seeds RH, et al. Reliability of reciprocal isokinetic testing of the knee exensors and flexors. J Orthop Sports Phys Ther 14(3): 121-127, 1991.

148. Li CK, Chan KM, Hsu SYC, et al. The Johnson antishear device and standard shin pad in the isokinetic assessment of the knee. Br J Sports Med 27(1): 49-52, 1993.

149. Li RCT, Chan KM, Hsu YC, et al. Isokinetic strength of the quadriceps and hamstrings and functional ability of anterior cruciate deficient knees in recreational athletes. Br J Sports Med, in print 1996.

150. Li RCT, Wu Y, Maffulli N, et al. Eccentric and concentric isokinetic knee flexion and extension: A reliability study using the Cybex 6000 dynamometer. Br J Sports Med, in print 1996.

151. Lieber RL. Skeletal muscle structure and function: Implications for rehabilitation and Sports Medicine 1992. Williams & Wilkins, London.

152. Lieber RL, Fridén J. Selective damage of fast glycolytic muscle fibers with eccentric contraction of the rabbit tibialis anterior. Acta Physiol Scand 133: 587-588, 1988.

153. Lindenfeld TN. The differentiation and treatment of ankle sprains. Sports Med 11(1): 203-206, 1988.

154. Lysens R, Steverlynck A, van den Auweele Y, et al. The predictability of sports injuries. Sports Med 1: 6-10, 1984.

155. MacDougall JD, Elder GCB, Sale DG, et al. Effects of strength training and immobilization on human muscle fibers. Eur J Appl Physiol 43: 25-34, 1980.

156. MacDougall JD, Tuxen D, Sale DG, et al. Arterial blood pressure response to heavy resistance exercise. J Appl Physiol 58: 785-790, 1985.

157. MacIntyre DL, Reid WD, McKenzie DC. Delayed muscle soreness: The inflammatory response to muscle injury and its clinical implications. Sports Med 20(1): 24-40, 1995.

158. Maffulli N, Binfield PM, King JB, et al. Acute hemarthrosis of the knee in athletes: A prospective study of 106 cases. J Bone Joint Surg (Br Vol) 75(B): 945-949, 1993.

159. Maffulli N, Pintore E. Intensive training in young athletes. Br J Sports Med 24(4): 237-239, 1990.

160. Magnusson SP, Gleim GW, Nicholas JA. Subject variability of shoulder abduction strength testing. Am J Sports Med 18(4): 349-353, 1990.

161. Mahler P, Mora C, Gremion G, et al. Isotonic muscle evaluation and sprint performance. Excel 8: 139-145, 1992.

162. Malerba JL, Adam ML, Harris BA, et al. Reliability of dynamic and isometric testing of shoulder external and internal rotators. J Orthop Sports Phys Ther 18(4): 543-552, 1993.

163. Marshall JL, Rubin RM. Knee ligament injuries: A diagnostic and therapeutic approach. Orthop Clin North Am 8: 641-668, 1977.

164. Marshall JL, Tischler HM. Screening for sports: Guidelines. New York State J Med 78: 243-251, 1978.

165. Mawdsley RH, Knapik JJ. Comparison of isokinetic measurements with test repetitions. Phys Ther 62(2): 169-172, 1982.

166. McCleary RW, Andersen JC. Test-re-test reliability of reciprocal isokinetic knee extension and flexion peak torque measurement. J Athletic Training 27(4): 362-365, 1992.

167. McCrory MA, Aitkens SG, Bernaurer EM. Reliability of concentric and eccentric measurements on the LIDO Active isokinetic dynamometer. Med Sci Sports Exerc [Abs] 21 (Suppl): S52, 1989.

168. McDaniel WJ, Dameron TB. The untreated anterior cruciate ligament rupture. Clin Orthop 172: 158-163, 1983.

169. McDonagh MJ, Hayward CM, Davies CT. Isometric training in human elbow flexor muscles: The effects on voluntary and electrically evoked forces. J Bone Joint Surg 65(3): 355-358, 1983.

170. McMaster WC, Long SC, Caiozzo VJ. Isokinetic torque imbalances in the rotator cuff of the elite water polo player. Am J Sports Med 19(1): 72-75, 1991.

171. Meadors WJ, Crews TR, Adeyanju K. A comparison of three conditioning protocols on the muscular strength and endurance of sedentary college women. Athletic Training 240: 242, 1983.

172. Mero A, Luhtanen P, Viitasalo JT, et al. Relationship between maximal running velocity, muscle fiber characteristics, force production and force relaxation of sprinters. Scand J Sports Sci 3: 16-22, 1981.

173. Moffroid MT, Whipple RH. Specificity of speed of exercise. J Orthop Sports Phys Ther 12(2): 72-78, 1990.

174. Moffroid M, Whipple R, Hofkosh J, et al. A study of isokinetic exercise. Phys Ther 49: 735-746, 1969.

175. Molczyk L, Thigpen LK, Eickhoff J, et al. Reliability of testing the knee extensors and flexors in healthy adult women using a Cybex II isokinetic dynamometer. J Orthop Sports Phys Ther 14(1): 37-41, 1991.

176. Molnar GE, Alexander J. Objective, quantitative muscle testing in children: A pilot study. Arch Phys Med Rehabil 54: 225-228, 1973.

177. Mont MA, Cohen DB, Campbell KR, et al. Isokinetic concentric versus eccentric training of shoulder rotators with functional evaluation of performance enhancement in elite tennis players. Am J Sports Med 22(4): 513-517, 1994.

178. Montgomery LC, Douglass LW, Deuster PA. Reliability of an isokinetic test of muscle strength and endurance. J Orthop Sports Phys Ther 10(8): 315-322, 1989.

179. Mookerjee S, Bibi KW, Kenney GA, et al. Relationship between isokinetic strength, flexibility, and flutter kicking speed in female collegiate swimmers. J Strength Conditioning Res 9(2): 71-74, 1995.

180. Morris JM, Lucas DB, Brester B. Role of the trunk in the stability of the spine. J Bone Joint Surg 43A: 327-351, 1961.

181. Morrissey MC, Harman EA, Johnson MJ. Resistance training modes: Specificity and effectiveness. Med Sci Sports Exerc 27(5): 648-660, 1995.

182. Moss CL, Wright P. Comparison of three methods of assessing muscle strength and imbalance ratios of the knee. J Athletic Training 28(1): 55-58, 1993.

183. Mulder HH. Ice hockey injuries. J Sports Med 1: 41-42, 1973.

184. Murray SM, Warren RF, Otis JC, et al. Torque-velocity relationships of the knee extensor and flexor muscles in individuals sustaining injuries of the anterior cruciate ligament. Am J Sports Med 12: 436-440, 1984.

185. Nakazawa K, Kawakami Y, Fukunaga T, et al. Differences in activation patterns in elbow flexors during isometric, concentric and eccentric contractions. Eur J Appl Physiol 66: 214-220, 1993.

186. National Research Institute of Sports Science. The physiological characteristics of elite swimmers in China. Selection of Research Papers 2: 19-31, 1988.

187. Nelson AJ, Moffroid M, Wipple R. The relationship of integrated electromyographic discharge to isokinetic contractions. In Desmedt JE (Ed) New Developments in Electromyographic and Clinical Neurophysiology 584-595, 1973. Karger, Basel.

188. Nisell R, Ericson MO, Nemeth G, et al. Tibiofemoral joint forces during isokinetic knee extension. Am J Sports Med 17: 49-54, 1989.

189. Norman RW, Komi PV. Electromyographic delay in skeletal muscle under normal movement conditions. Acta Physiol Scand 106: 241, 1979.

190. Nosse LJ. Assessment of selected reports on the strength relationship of the knee musculature. J Orthop Sports Phys Ther 4: 78-85, 1982.

191. Noyes FR, Mangine RE, Barber S. Early knee motion after open and arthroscopic anterior cruciate ligament reconstruction. Am J Sports Med 15(2): 149-160, 1987.

192. Nunn KD, Mayhew JL. Comparison of three methods of assessing strength imbalances at the knee. J Orthop Sports Phys Ther 10(4): 134-137, 1988.

193. O'Donoghue DH. Reconstruction for medial instability of the knee: Technique and results of 6 cases. J Bone Joint Surg 55A: 941-955, 1973.

194. O'Driscoll SW, Kumar A, Salter RB. The effect of continuous passive motion (CPM) on the clearance of a hemarthrosis from a synovial joint: An experimental investigation in the rabbit. Clin Orthop Related Res 176: 305-311, 1983.

195. Oberg B, Moller M, Gillquist J, et al. Isokinetic torque levels for knee extensors and knee flexors in soccer players. Int J Sports Med 7(1): 50-53, 1986.

196. Ohkoshi Y, Yasuda K, Kaneda K, et al. Biomechanical analysis of rehabilitation in the standing position. Am J Sports Med 19: 605-611, 1991.

197. Osternig LR. Isokinetic dynamometry: Implications for muscle testing and rehabilitation. Exerc Sports Sci Rev 14: 45-80, 1986.

198. Osternig LR, Hamill J, Sawhill JA, et al. Influence of torque and limb speed on power production in isokinetic exercise. Am J Phys Med 62: 163-171, 1983.

199. Palmieri GA. Weight training and repetition speed. J Appl Sport Sci Res 1: 36-38, 1987.

200. Palmitier RA, An KN, Scott SG, et al. Kinetic chain exercise in knee rehabilitation. Sports Med 11(6): 402-413, 1991.

201. Parker M. Calculation of isokinetic rehabilitation velocities for the knee extensors. J Orthop Sports Phys Ther 4: 32-35, 1982.

202. Paton RW, Grimshaw P, McGregor J, et al. Biomechanical assessment of the effects of significant hamstring injury: An isokinetic study. J Biomed Eng 11(3): 229-230, 1989.

203. Pauletto B. Strength training for coaches 164,1991. Leisure Press, Champaign.

204. Paulos L, Noyes FR, Grood E, et al. Knee rehabilitation after anterior cruciate ligament reconstruction and repair. Am J Sports Med 9: 140-147, 1981.

205. Pawlowski D, Perrin DH. Relationship between shoulder and elbow isokinetic peak torque, torque acceleration energy, average power, and total work and throwing velocity in intercollegiate pitchers. Athletic Training 24: 129-132, 1989.

206. Pearson DR, Costill DL. The effects of constant external resistance exercise and isokinetic exercise training on work-induced hypertrophy. J Appl Sport Sci Res 2: 39-41, 1988.

207. Perrin DH. Isokinetic Exercise and Assessment, 1993. Human Kinetics Publishers, Champaign.

208. Perrin DH. Reliability of isokinetic measures. Athletic Training 21: 319-321, 1986.

209. Perrin DH, Lephart SM, Weltman A. Specificity of training on computer obtained isokinetic measures. J Orthop Sports Phys Ther 11: 495-498, 1989.

210. Perrine JJ, Edgerton VR. Isokinetic anaerobic ergometry. Med Sci Sports 7: 79, 1975.

211. Petersen SR, Bagnall KM, Wenger HA, et al. The influence of velocity-specific resistance training on the in vivo torque-velocity relationship and the cross-sectional area of quadriceps femoris. J Orthop Sports Phys Ther 11: 456-462, 1989.

212. Peterson L, Renström PAFH. Sports injuries: Their prevention and treatment. Ed, 1986. Hope K. Martin Dunitz Ltd., London.

213. Pipes TV, Wilmore JH. Isokinetic vs isotonic strength training in adult men. Med Sci Sports 7(4): 262-274, 1975.

214. Pitetti KH. A reliable isokinetic strength test for arm and leg musculature for mildly mentally retarded adults. Arch Phys Med Rehabil 71: 669-673, 1990.

215. Posch E, Haglund Y, Eriksson E. Prospective study of concentric and eccentric leg muscle torques, flexibility, physical conditioning, and variation of injury rates during on season of amateur ice hockey. Int J Sports Med 10: 113, 1989.

216. Rantanen P, Penttinen E, Rinta-Kauppila S. Cardiovascular stress in isokinetic trunk strength test. Spine 20(4): 485-488, 1995.

217. Read MTF, Bellamy MJ. Comparison of hamstring/quadriceps isokinetic strength ratios and power in tennis, squash and track athletes. Br J Sports Med 24(3): 178-182, 1990.

218. Requa RK, DeAvilla LN, Garrick JG. Injuries in recreational adult fitness activities. Am J Sports Med 21: 461-467, 1993.

219. Richter KJ. Subcutaneous hemorrhage in a patient on coumadin: An isokinetic exercise complication. J Sport Rehabil 1: 264-266, 1992.

220. Rothstein JM, Lamb RL, Mayhew TP. Clinical uses of isokinetic measurements. Phys Ther 67: 1840-1844, 1987.

221. Ryan LM, Magidow PS, Duncan PW. Velocity-specific and mode-specific effects of eccentric isokinetic training of the hamstrings. J Orthop Sports Phys Ther 13: 33-39, 1991.

222. Sale DG. Neural adaptations to strength training. In Komi PV (Ed) Strength and Power in Sport 249-265, 1992. Blackwell Scientific Publications, London.

223. Sale DG, Moroz DE, McKelvie RS. Comparison of blood pressure response to isokinetic and weightlifting exercise. Eur J Appl Physiol 67(2): 115-120, 1993.

224. Salter RB, Simmonds DF, Malcolm BW, et al. The biological effects of continuous passive motion on the healing of full-thickness defects in articular cartilage. J Bone Joint Sur 62A(8): 1232-1251, 1980.

225. Sandberg R, Balkfors B. The durability of anterior cruciate ligament reconstruction with the patellar tendon. Am J Sports Med 4: 341-343, 1988.

226. Sapega AA. Current concepts review: Muscle performance evaluation in orthopedic practice. J Bone Joint Surg 72A(10): 1562-1574, 1990.

227. Sapega AA, Minkoff J, Nicholas JA, et al. Sport-specific performance factor profiling. Am J Sports Med 6(5): 232-235, 1978.

228. Scharf HP, Eckhardt R, Maurus M, et al. Metabolic and hemodynamic changes during isokinetic muscle training: A controlled clinical trial. Int J Sports Med 15: S56-S59, 1994.

229. Schlinkman B. Norms for high school football players derived from Cybex data reduction computer. J Orthop Sports Phys Ther 5: 243-254, 1984.

230. Shelbourne KD, Nitz P. Accelerated rehabilitation after anterior cruciate ligament reconstruction. Am J Sports Med 18(3): 292-299, 1990.

231. Sherman WM, Pearson DR, Plyley MJ, et al. Isokinetic rehabilitation after surgery: A review of factors which are important for developing physiotherapeutic techniques after knee surgery. Am J Sports Med 10(3): 155-161, 1982.

232. Slagle GW. The importance of pretesting the knee joint. Athletic Training 14: 225-226, 1979.

233. Sleivert GG, Wenger HA. Reliability of measuring isometric and isokinetic peak torque, rate of torque development, integrated electromyography, and tibial nerve conduction velocity. Arch Phys Med Rehabil 75: 1315-1321, 1994.

234. Smidt GL, Amundsen LR, Dostal WF. Muscle strength at the trunk. J Orthop Sports Phys Ther 1(3): 165-170, 1980.

235. Smidt GL, Herring T, Amundsen L, et al. Assessment of abdominal and back extensor function: A quantitative approach and results for chronic low back patients. Spine 8: 211-219, 1983.

236. Smith DJ, Quinney HA, Wenger HA, et al. Isokinetic torque outputs of professional and elite amateur ice hockey players. J Orthop Sports Phys Ther 3(2): 42-47, 1981.

237. Smith MJ, Melton P. Isokinetic versus isotonic variable-resistance training. Am J Sports Med 9: 275-279, 1981.

238. Smith RW, Reischl SF. Treatment of ankle sprains in young athletes. Am J Sports Med 14(6): 465-471, 1986.

239. Snow CJ, Blacklin K. Reliability of knee flexor peak torque measurement from a standardized test protocol on a Kin-Com dynamometer. Arch Phys Med Rehabil 73: 15-21, 1992.

240. So RC, Siu OT, Chin MK, et al. Bilateral isokinetic variables of the shoulder: A prediction model for young men. Br J Sports Med 29(2): 105-109, 1995.

241. Solomonow M, Baratta R, Zhou BH, et al. The synergistic action of the anterior cruciate ligament and thigh muscles in maintaining joint stability. Am J Sports Med 15(3): 207-213, 1987.

242. Stanish WD, Rubinovich RM, Curwin S. Eccentric exercise in chronic tendinitis. Clin Orthop Related Res 208: 65-68, 1986.

243. Stanton P, Purdam C. Hamstring injuries in sprinting: The role of eccentric exercise. J Orthop Sports Phys Ther 10(9): 343-349, 1989.

244. Steiner LA, Harris BA, Krebs DE. Reliability of eccentric isokinetic knee flexion and extension measurements. Arch Phys Med Rehabil 74: 1327-1335, 1993.

245. Stewart K. Conditioning for tennis.in: Some basic consideration toward an understanding of human performance. 262-266, 1977. Movement Publications, Ithaca, NY.

246. Suomi R, Surburg PR, Lecius P. Reliability of isokinetic and isometric measurement of leg strength on men with mental retardation. Arch Phys Med Rehabil 74:848-852, 1993.

247. Tegner Y, Lysholm J, Lysholm M, et al. A performance test to monitor rehabilitation and evaluate anterior cruciate ligament injuries. Am J Sports Med 14: 156-159, 1986.

248. Thigpen LK, Blanke D, Lang P. The reliability of two different Cybex isokinetic systems. J Orthop Sports Phys Ther 12(4): 157-162, 1990.

249. Thistle HG, Hislop HJ, Moffroid M, et al. Isokinetic contraction: A new concept of resisted exercise. Arch Phys Med Rehabil 48: 279-282, 1967.

250. Thorstensson A, Grimby G, Karlsson J. Force-velocity relations and fiber composition in human knee extensor muscles. J Appl Physiol 40: 12-16, 1976.

251. Timm KE. Postsurgical knee rehabilitation: A 5-year study of 4 methods and 5,381 patients. Am J Sports Med 16(5): 463-468, 1988.

252. Timm KE. Investigation of the physiological overflow effect from speed-specific isokinetic activity. J Orthop Sports Phys Ther 9(3): 106-110, 1987.

253. Timm KE. Validation of the Johnson anti-shear accessory as an accurate and effective clinical isokinetic instrument. J Orthop Sports Phys Ther 7: 198-303, 1986.

254. Tomberlin JP, Basford JR, Schwen EE, et al. Comparative study of isokinetic eccentric and concentric quadriceps training. J Orthop Sports Phys Ther 14: 31-36, 1991.

255. Tredinnick TJ, Duncan PW. Reliability of measurements of concentric and eccentric isokinetic loading. Phys Ther 68: 656-659, 1988.

256. Tripp EJ, Harris SR. Test-re-test reliability of isokinetic knee extension and flexion torque measurements in persons withh spastic hemiparesis. Phys Ther 71(5): 390-396, 1991.

257. Trudell-Jackson E, Meske N, Highenboten C, et al. Eccentric/concentric torque deficits in the quadriceps muscle. J Orthop Sports Phys Ther 11: 142-145, 1989.

258. Tupling SJ, Davis GM. Wheelchair impulse generation and arm strength in the physically disabled. Can J Appl Sports Sci 8: 228, 1983.

259. Urquhart DS, Garbutt G, Cova K, et al. Isokinetics: Applications in the management of knee soft-tissue injuries. Sports Exerc Injury 1: 138-147, 1995.

260. Van Oteghen SL. Two speeds of isokinetic exercise as related to the vertical jump performance of women. Res Q Exerc Sport 46: 78-84, 1973.

261. Vegso JJ, Genuario SE, Torg JS. Maintenance of hamstrings strength following knee surgery. Med Sci Sports Exerc 17: 376-379, 1985.

262. Verdonck A, Frobose I, Hardelauf U, et al. Contraction patterns during isokinetic eccentric and concentric contractions after anterior cruciate ligament injury. Int J Sports Med 15 (Suppl 1): S60-S63, 1994.

263. Viitasalo JT, Aura O. Seasonal fluctuations of force production in high jumpers. Can J Appl Sport Sci 9: 209-213, 1984.

264. Viitasalo JT, Häkkinen K, Komi PV. Isometric and dynamic force production and muscle fiber composition in man. J Human Movement Studies 7: 199-209, 1981.

265. Walsh WM, Blackburn T. Prevention of ankle sprains. Am J Sport Med 5(6): 243-245, 1997.

266. Warner JJP, Micheli LJ, Arslania LE, et al. Patterns of flexibility, laxity and strength in normal shoulders and shoulders with instability and impingement. Am J Sports Med 18(4): 366-375, 1990.

267. Wathen D. Muscle balance. In Baech TR(Ed) Essentials of strength training and conditioning 424-428, 1994. National Strength and Conditioning Association. Human Kinetics Publishers, Champaign.

268. Watkins PM, Harris AB, Kozlowski BA. Isokinetic training in patients with hemiparesis. Phys Ther 64: 184-189, 1984.

269. Weir JP, Wagner LL, Housh TJ. Linearity and reliability of the IEMG torque relationship for the forearm flexors and leg extensors. Am J Phys Med Rehabil 71(5): 283-287, 1992.

270. Wennerberg D. Reliability of an isokinetic dorsiflexion and plantarflexion apparatus. Am J Sports Med 19: 519-522, 1991.

271. Wessel J, Ford D, Van Driesum D. Measurement of torque of trunk flexors at different velocities. Scand J Rehabil 24:175-180, 1992.

272. Wessel J, Mattison G, Luongo F, et al. Reliability of eccentric and concentric measurements. Phys Ther 68: 782, 1988.

273. Westing SH, Seger JY. Eccentric and concentric torque-velocity characteristics, torque output comparisons, and gravity effect torque corrections for the quadriceps and hamstring muscles in females. Int J Sports Med 10: 175-180, 1989.

274. Wiklander J, Lysholm J. Simple tests for surveying muscle strength and muscle stiffness in sportsmen. Int J Sports Med 8: 50-54, 1987.

275. Wilhite MR, Cohen ER, Wilhite SC. Reliability of concentric and eccentric measurements of quadriceps performance using the Kin-Com dynamometer: The effect of testing order for three different speeds. J Orthop Sports Phys Ther 15: 175-182, 1992.

276. Wilmore JH. Letter to the editor. Med Sci Sports Exerc 2: iii, 1979.

277. Wilson G, Murphy A. The efficacy of isokinetic, isometric and vertical jump tests in exercise science. Aust J Sci Med Sport 27(1): 20-24, 1995.

278. Winter DA, Wells RP, Orr GW. Errors in the use of isokinetic dynamometers. Eur J Appl Physiol 46: 397-408, 1981.

279. Wong JPS. Isokinetic profile of trunk muscles in athletes: A quantitative study with correlation to sports performance. MPhil thesis, 1994. The Chinese University of Hong Kong.

280. Worrell TW, Perrirn DH, Gansneder B, et al. Comparison of isokinetic strength and flexibility measures between hamstrings injured and non-injured athletes. J Orthop Sport Phys Ther 13:118-125, 1991.

281. Wyse JP, Mercer TH, Gleeson NP. Time-of-day dependence of isokinetic leg strength and associated interday variability. Br J Sports Med 28(3): 167-170, 1994.

282. Yack HJ, Collins CE, Whieldon TJ. Comparison of closed and open kinetic chain exercise in the anterior cruciate ligament-deficient knee. Am J Sports Med 21: 49-54, 1993.

283. Yeung MS, Chan KM, So CH, et al. An epidemiological survey on ankle sprain. Br J Sports Med 28(2): 112-116, 1994

284. Yeung MSJ. Isokinetic rehabilitation of ankle sprain. MPhil thesis, 1992. The Chinese University of Hong Kong.

285. Young WB, Bilby GE. The effect of voluntary effort to influence speed of contraction on strength, muscular power, and hypertrophy development. J Strength Conditioning Res. 7: 172-178, 1993.

Further Readings

1.   Appen L, Duncan WP. Strength relationship of the knee musculature: Effect of gravity and sport. J Orthop Sports Phys Ther 7:232-235, 1986.

2.   Baltzopoulos V, Brodie DA. Isokinetic dynamometry: Applications and limitations. Sports Med 8: 101-116, 1989.

3.   Baltzopoulos V, Brodie DA. The development of a computer system for real time display and analysis of isokinetic data. Clin Biomech 4: 118-120, 1989.

4.   Barbee J, Landis D. Reliability of Cybex computer measures [Abs]. Phys Ther 64: 737, 1984.

5.   Bemben M, Grump K, Massey B. Assessment of technical accuracy of the Cybex II isokinetic dynamometer and analog recording system. J Orthop Sports Phys Ther 10:12-17, 1988.

6.   Best TM, Garrett WE. Muscle-tendon unit injuries. In Renström PAFH (Ed) Sports Injuries: Basic Principles of Prevention and Care 71-86, 1993. Blackwell Scientific Publications, London.

7.   Brown LP, Niehues SL, Harrah A, et al. Upper extremity range of motion and isokinetic strength of the internal and external shoulder rotators in major league baseball players. Am J Sports Med 16: 577-585, 1988.

8.   Cetti R, Christensen SE, Corfitzen MT. Ruptured fibular ankle ligament: Plaster or pliton brace? Br J Sports Med 18(2): 104-109, 1984.

9.   Cybex 6000 Testing and Rehabilitation System Users Guide, 1991-1993. CYBEX Division of LUNEX, Inc. Ronkonkoma, NY.

10. Edman DAP. Contractile performance of skeletal muscle fibers. In Komi PV (Ed) Strength and Power in Sport 96-114, 1992. Blackwell Scientific Publications, London.

11. Fillyaw M, Bevins T, Fernandez L. Importance of correcting isokinetic peak joint moment for the effect of gravity when calculating knee flexor to extensor muscle ratios. Phys Ther 66: 23-31, 1986.

12. Francis K, Hoobler T. Comparison of peak torque values of the knee flexor and extensor muscle groups using the Cybex II and LIDO 2.0 isokinetic dynamometers. J Orthop Sports Phys Ther 8: 480-483, 1987.

13. Gross MT, Huffman GM, Phillips CN, et al. Intramachine and intermachine reliability of the Biodex and Cybex II for knee flexion and extension peak torque and angular work. J Orthop Sports Phys Ther 13: 329-335, 1991.

14. Hanten WP, Ramberg CL. Effect of stabilization on maximal isokinetic torque of the quadriceps femoris muscle during concentric and eccentric contractions. Phys Ther 68(2): 219-222, 1988.

15. Harris UJ, Bassey EJ. Torque-velocity relationship for the knee extensors in women in their third and seventh decades. Eur J Appl Physiol 60: 187-190,1990.

16. Herzog W. The relation between the resultant moments at a joint and the moments measured by an isokinetic dynamometer. J Biomechnaics 21: 5-12, 1988.

17. Hinson M, Smith W, Funk S. Isokinetics: A clarification. Res Q 50:30-35, 1979.

18. Hortobagyi T, Katch FI. Reliability of muscle mechanical characteristics for isokinetic squat and bench exercise using a multifunction computerized dynamometer. Res Q Exerc Sports 16: 191-195, 1990.

19. Knuttgen HG, Komi PV. Basic definitions for exercise. In Komi PV (Ed) Strength and Power in Sport 3-6, 1992. Blackwell Scientific Publications, London.

20. Kramer JF, Hill K, Jones IC, et al. Effect of dynamometer application arm length on concentric and eccentric torques during isokinetic knee extension. Physiotherapy Canada 41: 100-106, 1989.

21. Lewin G. The incidence of injury in an English professional soccer club during one competitive season. Physiotherapy 75(10): 601-605, 1989.

22. Li R. Anterior cruciate ligament deficiency: A functional and clinical correlation. MPhil Thesis, 1989. The Chinese University of Hong Kong.

23. LIDO Active isokinetic rehabilitation system manual, 1989. Loredan Biomedical Incorporated. Davis, CA, USA.

24. Lo C. Shoulder impingement syndrome: A pilot study on epidemiology and prevention. MPhil Thesis, 1990. The Chinese University of Hong Kong.

25. Lumex Inc: The Cybex 6000 extremity system product information brochure 4-40, 1991. Ronkonkoma, NY: Cybex.

26. MacIntyre DL, Wessel J. Knee muscle torques in patellofemoral pain syndrome. Physiotherapy Canada 40: 20-24, 1988.

27. Murray D. Optimal filtering of constant velocity torque data. Med Sci Sports Exerc 18: 603-611, 1986.

28. Murray DA, Harrison E. Constant velocity dynamometry: An appraisal using mechanical loading. Med Sci Sports Exerc 18:612-624, 1986.

29. Nelson S, Duncan P. Correction of isokinetic torque recordings for the effect of gravity. Phys Ther 63:674-676, 1983.

30. Nisell R, Ericson MO, Nemeth G, et al. Tibiofemoral joint forces during isokinetic knee extension. Am J Sports Med 17:49-54,1989.

31. Nisell R. Nemeth G, Ohlsen H. Joint forces in extension of the knee. Acta Orthop Scand 57:41-46, 1986.

32. Osternig LR, Hamill J, Lander J, et al. Co-activation patterns of sprinter and distance runner agonist/ antagonist muscles in isokinetic exercise [Abs]. Med Sci Sports Exerc 17: 248, 1985.

33. Osternig LR, Hamill J, Lander JE, et al. Co-activation of sprinter and distance runner muscle in isokinetic exercise. Med Sci Sports Exerc 18(4): 431-435, 1986.

34. Osternig LR, Sawhill JA, Bates BT, et al. Function of limb speed on torque patterns of antagonist muscles. In Biomechanics VIII-A, 1983. Human Kinetics Publishers, Champaign.

35. Patterson LA, Spivey WE. Validity and reliability of the LIDO Active isokinetic dynamometer. J Orthop Sports Phys Ther 15: 32-36, 1992.

36. Pedegana LR, Elsner R, Roberts D, et al. The relationship of upper extremity strength to throwing speed. Am J Sports Med 10: 352-354, 1982.

37. Perrin DH, Robertson RJ, Ray RL. Bilateral isokinetic peak torque, torque acceleration energy, power, and work relationships in athletes and non-athletes. J Orthop Sports Phys Ther 9: 184-189, 1987.

38. Renström PAFH (Ed) Sports Injuries: Basic Principles of Prevention and Care, 1993. Blackwell Scientific Publications, London.

39. Rizzardo M, Wessel J, Bay G. Eccentric and concentric torque and power of the knee extensors of females. Can J Sports Sci 13: 166-169, 1988.

40. Sale DG, MacDougall JD, Upton ARM, et al. Effect of strength training upon motoneuron excitability in man. Med Sci Sports Exerc 15(1): 57-62, 1983.

41. Sapega A, Nicholas J, Sokolow D, et al. The nature of torque "overshoot" in Cybex isokinetic dynamometry. Med Sci Sports Exerc 14: 368-375, 1982.

42. Sawhill JA, Bates BT, Osternig LR, et al. Variability of isokinetic measures. Med Sci Sports Exerc 14: 177, 1982.

43. Sinacore D, Rothstein J, Delitto A, et al. Effect of damp on isokinetic measurements. Phys Ther 63:1248-1250, 1983.

44. Snow C, Johnson K. Reliability of two velocity-controlled tests for the measurement of peak torque of the knee flexors during resisted muscle shortening and resisted muscle lengthening [Abs]. Phys Ther 68: 781, 1988.

45. So RCH. Isokinetic assessment musculoskeletal parameters in elite athletes. MPhil Thesis, 1993 The Chinese University of Hong Kong.

46. Thompson MC, Shingleton LG, Kegerreis ST. Comparison of values generated during testing of the knee using the Cybex II+ and Biodex model B 2000 isokinetic dynamometers. J Orthop Sports Phys Ther 11: 108-115, 1989.

47. Wilk KE, Andrews JR, Arrigo CA, et al. The internal and external rotator strength characteristics of professional baseball pitchers. Am J Sports Med 21: 61-66, 1993.

48. Winter DA, Wells RP, Orr GW. Errors in the use of isokinetic dynamometers. Eur J Appl Physiol 46:397-408, 1981.

49. Yeung MSJ. Isokinetic rehabilitation of ankle sprain. MPhil Thesis, 1992. The Chinese University of Hong Kong.

Subject Index

A

Absolute contraindications 116
Acceleration 120
ACL 47, 55
ACL reconstruction 120
ACL surgery 53
ACLI 126, 136
Actin filaments 2
Active dynamometers 13
Active mode 13
Acute sprain 116
Adaptation 47, 59, 63, 64
Age 40
Agonist 31, 112
Agonist/antagonist 111
Agonist/antagonist coactivation 35
Agonist/antagonist cycle 121
Agonist/antagonist ratios 18, 32, 36, 37, 172
Agonist muscle group 38, 112
AKP 43, 128, 160
Anaerobic threshold 91
Angle of occurrence 112
Angle of testing 34
Angle-specific torque 60, 112
Angular joint velocities 15
Angular velocity 11, 13, 33, 41, 83, 140
Ankle 15, 29
Ankle dorsiflexion 142
Ankle dorsiflexion/plantarflexion 32,120
Ankle eversion/inversion 32
Ankle inversion injury 141
Ankle joint 141
Ankle rehabilitation 144
Ankle sprain 141, 142
Antagonist 31, 38
Antagonist coactivation 35
Antagonist muscle group 112
Anterior cruciate ligament insufficiency 126
Anterior knee pain 11, 43, 57, 128, 160
Anterior tibial translation 56
Antishear device 140
AP 140, 175, 176
Articular cartilage 130

Assessment 134, 136, 141, 142, 146, 155, 160, 162
AST 60, 62
Asymmetrical activities 40
Asymmetry 37, 68
Athletic training 15
Atrophy 45, 47, 54, 136, 145
Average force 60, 62
Average power 113, 172, 182
Average work 182

B

Back 148
Back flexion/extension 32
Ballistic 83
Best work repetition 113
Bilateral 111
Bilateral comparison 175, 176
Bilateral deficit 73
Bilateral differences 18
Bilateral discrepancy 31, 37
Bilateral muscle strength 41
Bilateral strength 53
Biochemical adaptations 64
Biomechanical 93
Body composition 67
Body positioning 117
BWR 113

C

Calisthenics 53
Cardiovascular 147
CKC 54,76, 87
Closed kinetic chain 54, 84
Coactivation 55
Co-contraction 35, 84
Compression 54
Compressive 55, 140
Concentric 41, 59, 86, 110, 117, 120
Concentric action 5, 13, 14
Concentric contraction 38
Concentric/eccentric actions 121

Concentric exercise 57
Concentric flexion/extension 121
Concentric force 14
Concentric strength 39, 64
Contractures 45
Contraindications 115
Contralateral 36
Control of speed 13
CPM 10, 13, 16, 45, 87, 97, 134
Cross-sectional area 63, 111

D

Damage 16
Damping 13
Deceleration 38
Delayed muscle soreness 92
Delayed onset of muscle soreness 5
DF/PF 143
Diagnosis 11, 43, 97
Dislocation 116
Distance runners 35
Dominant 175, 176
Dominant arm 38
Dominant limb 119
Dominant side 37, 177
DOMS 5
Dynamic muscle strength 2
Dynamic performance 9
Dynamic variable-resistance mode 7

E

Eccentric 59, 86, 93, 110, 120
Eccentric action 5, 13, 117
Eccentric activation 87
Eccentric antagonist/concentric agonist ratio 40
Eccentric/concentric ratio 31, 38, 93
Eccentric force 14
Eccentric isokinetic training 64
Eccentric mode 16
Eccentric muscle strength 39
Eccentric strength 37
Eccentric training 39, 56, 62, 64, 92
Eccentric work 38
Eccentrically 41
Elbow 177

Elbow extension/flexion 76
Electromyography 2, 91
EMG 2, 47, 56
Endurance 3, 6, 10, 31, 32, 41, 64, 67, 74, 91, 93, 102, 112, 121, 139, 140, 172, 177
Endurance athletes 112
Endurance indices 114
Endurance ratio 114, 182
Explosive power 6, 114
Explosive sports 112
Explosiveness 10
Extension curve 128
Extension to flexion PT ratio 175

F

Familiarization 117
Fast fibers 40, 112
Fast muscle fibers 15
Fatigue index 3
Fatigue ratio 18
Fiber types 83
Flexibility 41, 67, 154
Flexion curve 128
Force 11, 35, 129
Force-generating capacity 111
Fractures 116
Frozen shoulder 132, 158
Functional ability 84, 140
Functional capacity 92
Functional movements 91
Functional performance 58, 62, 65
Functional rating scale 142
Functional score 140

G

Gender 40
General muscle weakness 31
General weakness 129
Gravity 32, 33, 38
Gravity control 16
Gravity correction 3, 40, 120
Gravity-loaded system 10

Resistance training 15
Rest 121
Reversibility 58
ROM 44, 45, 112, 120, 121, 129, 132, 144, 158

S

Safe 56
Safety 15
Screening 31
Sexes 80
Shear forces 55, 140
Shin pad 140
Shoulder 15, 23, 28
Shoulder abduction/adduction 32
Shoulder extension 32, 37, 76, 177
Shoulder external rotation 32, 33, 76, 120
Shoulder external rotators 73
Shoulder flexion 32, 37
Shoulder flexors 177
Shoulder horizontal adduction 76
Shoulder horizontal abduction/adduction 177
Shoulder impingement 42, 130
Shoulder impingement syndromes 155
Shoulder internal/external rotator ratio 37
Shoulder internal rotation 32, 33, 76, 120
Shoulder internal rotators 38, 73
SIR/SER 37
Slow fiber 45
Slow muscle fibers 15
Soft-tissue injury 15
Specificity 53, 58
Speed 56, 80, 175
Speed specificity 60, 62
Spinal surgery 147
Sports Medicine 87, 102, 103
Sports-specific 93
Sprinters 35
SSC 5
Stabilization 119, 125, 138, 144
Standardized 122
Strains 13
Strength 6, 32, 41, 67, 102
Strength assessment 87
Strength imbalance 32
Strength overflows 14
Strength training 47, 57

Stress fracture 130
Stretch-shortening cycle 5, 87
Stretching 117
Subacromial bursitis 132
Subluxation 116
Submaximal 121
Surgery 13, 32
Symmetry 38

T

Tears 13
Tendinitis 53, 57, 133
Tendonitis 43
Test angle 32
Test order 139
Test speed 177
Test velocities 14
Testing protocol 120, 137, 148, 155, 158
Tightness 141
Time rate of tension development 127
Time to peak torque 112
Tissue healing 53
Torque 6, 10, 11, 22, 31, 35, 37, 39, 40, 43, 56, 63, 68, 110, 120
Torque channel 13
Torque limits 15
Torque stylus 13
Torque-velocity ratio 112
Total work 3, 113, 172, 182
Training 11, 54, 60, 82, 91, 154
Training effect 120
Training speed 53
Training status 40
Training velocity 61
Treatment 97
Trick movements 121
TRTD 127
Trunk 15, 28, 146, 148
Trunk extension/flexion 77, 120
Trunk extensor 29
TW 140, 175, 176

U

UBXT 22
Unaffected limb 119

Uninjured limbs 141
Upper body exercise table 22

V

Validity 22, 37, 91
Variability 80
Velocity 32, 120, 121, 144
Velocity spectrum 64
Velocity spectrum training 15, 154
Verbal encouragement 122
Visual feedback 122

W

Warm-up 117, 120, 121
Weakness 141
Weight-bearing 32, 54, 55, 56, 112, 119, 120
Weight training 58, 63
Work 6, 10, 22, 40, 76, 182
Work ratio 172
Wrist 29